THE
BODY SHAPING DIET

THE
BODY SHAPING DIET

SANDRA CABOT MD

First published in 1993 by WHAS Pty. Ltd. Australia.
Reprinted 12 times
First published by SCB International Incorporated August 2000. USA
© Dr Sandra Cabot

Contact details for Dr Sandra Cabot
P.O.Box 5070
Glendale AZ 85312–5070–USA
Phone: 1888 75 LIVER or 623 3343232
Email: cabot@ozemail.com.au
Websites
www.weightcontroldoctor.com
www.liverdoctor.com
www.sandracabot.com

Dr Cabot, Sandra
The Body Shaping Diet.

Includes index.
ISBN 0-9673983-5-5

1. Diet. 2. Women–Health and hygiene. 3. Exercise for women. 4. Women–Nutrition. I. II. Title.

613.7045

Printed by Griffin Press

CONTENTS

DEDICATION

This book is dedicated to the late Vicki Petersen, undoubtedly the most brilliant and witty Australian health writer I have ever known. For those who were fortunate enough to know Vicki life will never be the same. I first met her in Sydney in 1981, when I was starting to put pen to paper. She was at this time a prolific journalist for many top women's magazines including *Vogue, Harper's Bazaar, Nature and Health and Woman's Day* and wrote with such panache and enthusiasm that one could always recognise the typical stamp of a Petersen article.

She had written several international best-selling books including *Whole Food Catalogue, Eat Your Way to Health, Strategies of the Champions, Food Combining* and a travel book on Australia and had so many plans to write future books on health and well-being, the next one off the press was to be a cookbook called *The Lean Green Mamma's Cookbook* and *Be Happy Not Hungry*.

Whoever would have thought that this brilliant and powerful woman was to become a victim of anorexia nervosa.

It came as a huge shock to all who knew and read her when she died in one of Sydney's public hospitals on the 29 August 1992, with kidney and liver failure as a result of malnutrition.

It is a tragedy that it takes the untimely death of such a tremendous woman as Vicki Petersen to bring home the message that we need to do more to help women with eating disorders. We need to do more for women caught in the lonely battle against eating disorders and obesity and the associated chronic health problems and dangers that they incur. We can change our body weight and shape in a scientific, safe and enjoyable way without becoming neurotically unhappy and caught in the superficial and stereotyped expectations that today's society projects. Obesity and eating disorders are a state of mind reflecting a loss of balance in our mental, emotional and physical lives. They are not primarily a physical disease such as a cold or arthritis which can be alleviated by treating the symptoms. We need to dig deeper and find the hidden mental agenda of negativity, poor self-image and loss of confidence.

The book *The Body Shaping Diet* has been written to overcome these negative aspects in our mind that keep us trapped in obesity or an eating disorder. It is not just another 'hip and thigh diet', but rather a way of eating for a vital mind and body. *The Body Shaping Diet* will re-balance your hormonal and metabolic system specifically for your body shape. It will stimulate your entire physical and mental physiology increasing your energy levels and vitality, thus overcoming all the negative obstacles in your mind that have previously held you back and told you that you cannot be slim and healthy and feel good about yourself. You no longer have to feel that you are alone in your struggle to maintain a healthy body weight because Dr Sandra Cabot has written this book as a vehicle to travel with you and guide and support you in your journey to total health.

ABOUT THE AUTHOR

Dr Sandra Cabot MBBS, DRCOG is a medical doctor who has extensive clinical experience in helping women with weight problems, hormonal disorders and chronic health problems. A member of the Australian Council for Responsible Nutrition, she has helped many thousands of women through her several books, The Liver Cleansing Diet, The Healthy Liver and Bowel Book, Menopause-HRT and its Natural Alternatives and Boost your Energy, which are self-help guides explaining the tremendous power of nutritional medicine and natural hormone therapy.

THE FOUR BODY TYPES

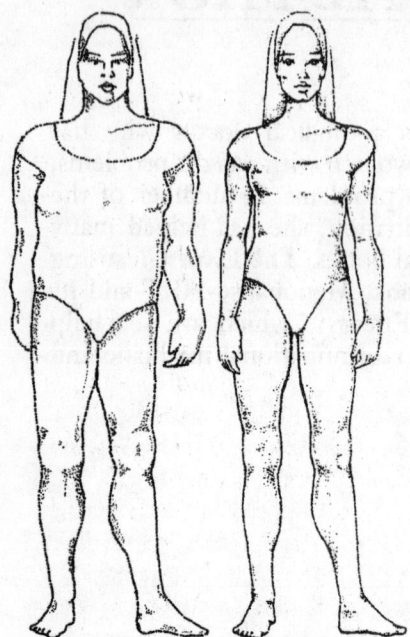

Android body shape (left) overweight, (right) ideal weight

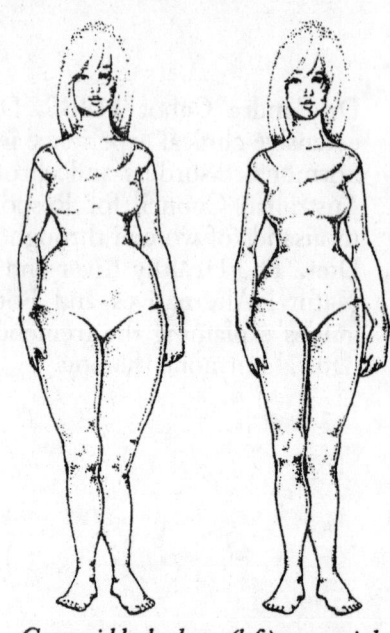

Gynaeoid body shape (left) overweight, (right) ideal weight

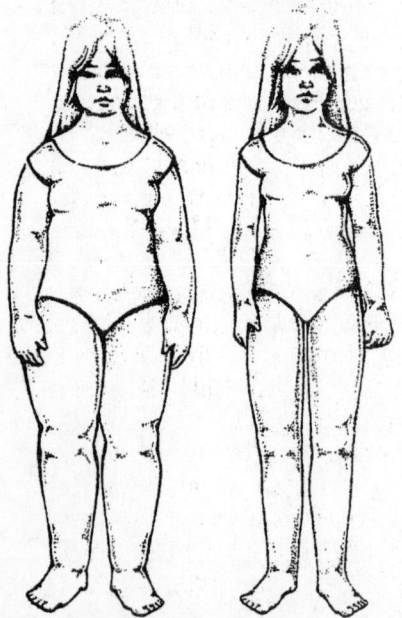

Lymphatic body shape (left) overweight, (right) ideal weight

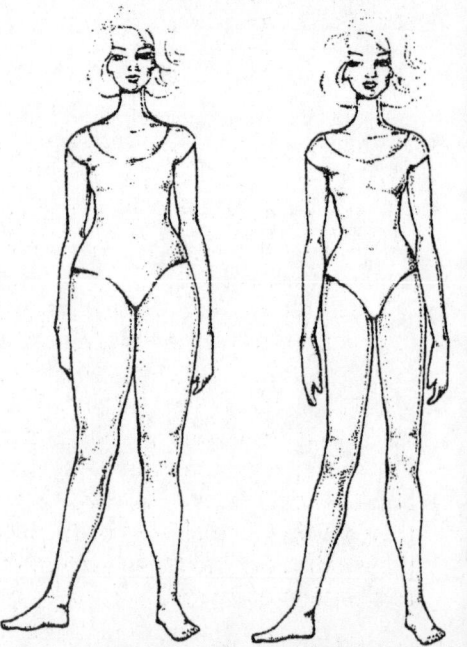

Thyroid body shape (left) overweight, (right) ideal weight

INTRODUCTION

The last twenty five years of my life have been spent working with women suffering with chronic health problems, hormonal imbalance and excess weight. I have researched these areas extensively and have a vast experience in investigating and treating women in a clinical context. Thanks to technology and sophisticated tools of diagnosis, it is now easy to scientifically pinpoint the type of hormonal imbalance present. We can now tell from blood hormone assays whether your numerous glands, such as the pituitary, thyroid, adrenals and ovaries, are under or overactive. It is possible to treat these imbalances with hormone replacement therapy using natural types of hormones and for this we can lay our gratitude firmly at the door of modern medicine.

However, when it comes to a large array of chronic health complaints, weight excess being included here, the tools of modern medicine, and chemical pharmacology often provide only partial or temporary solutions. Thankfully, for the last twenty years I have researched nutritional medicine, an interest of mine which started way back in medical school. The science and art of treating diseases and obesity with special diets, vitamins, minerals, amino acids and essential fatty acids is a tremendously satisfying healing tool for any doctor. It is a form of healing that I am able to utilise and write about with authority because of my background and my years of clinical experience with thousands of patients who were not responding to conventional medicine alone. If you are battling with a weight problems and its associated health complaints, I assure you that you can overcome them with a change of diet and specific nutritional strategies—all it takes is the decision to start. Make it today! The first three months is the hardest phase but after six months you will be feeling and looking much better and after twelve months on the Body Shaping Diet you will feel and look the best you can possibly be!

The Body Shaping Diet has been followed by many of my patients for many different reasons. Some have used it to lower their blood pressure, eradicate candida and allergies, reduce headaches or to improve their general health. Others have used it just to lose weight while some have stuck to it for years in a committed effort to change their body shape. No one has a perfect body and we all have room for improvement. Some women become really 'hung up' or unhappy about a part of themselves, so much so that they allow it to erode their self-esteem and personality. I try to show women that they must first accept themselves as a unique individual with a unique beauty. The next step is to make

Diagram 1

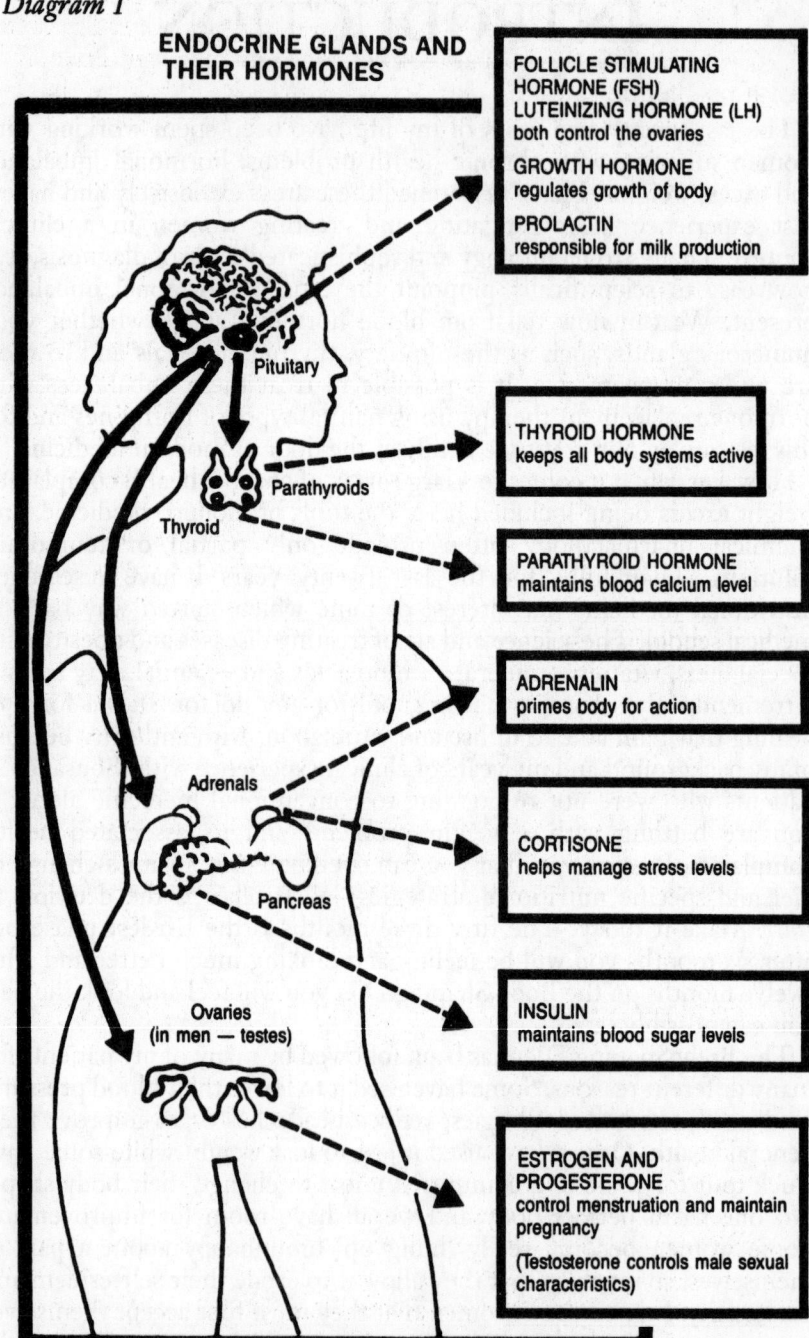

ENDOCRINE GLANDS AND THEIR HORMONES

FOLLICLE STIMULATING HORMONE (FSH)
LUTEINIZING HORMONE (LH)
both control the ovaries

GROWTH HORMONE
regulates growth of body

PROLACTIN
responsible for milk production

THYROID HORMONE
keeps all body systems active

PARATHYROID HORMONE
maintains blood calcium level

ADRENALIN
primes body for action

CORTISONE
helps manage stress levels

INSULIN
maintains blood sugar levels

ESTROGEN AND PROGESTERONE
control menstruation and maintain pregnancy

(Testosterone controls male sexual characteristics)

Pituitary

Parathyroids

Thyroid

Adrenals

Pancreas

Ovaries
(in men — testes)

the best of what you've got right now, today! Don't let life pass you by! You should never change yourself just to please another but rather do it first for yourself. The Body Shaping Diet and exercise programmes will make it possible for you to achieve your desired weight or to change your shape if you wish, so that you can feel really great about being you. Whether you want to look sexier, fitter, slimmer, more sporty, more or less shapely or simply glow with health the Body Shaping Diet can do it for you.

WHAT IS THE BODY SHAPING DIET?

It is a unique and specifically designed eating plan for life. There are four different eating plans specifically tailored for the four different body shapes of women. All women fall into one of these four categories - gynaeoid, android, thyroid and lymphatic - which you will understand as you read this book (see page 19). Each of the four body shapes, if exposed to the wrong types of foods on a consistent basis, may become obese in different areas of their body. Some body shapes can eat so-called 'fattening foods' without becoming obese while other body shapes cannot. Similarly, no one simple calorie restricted diet works for all body shapes and it is more important to change the sources of the calories than to just restrict them. These difference apply because each body shape has a unique metabolic and hormonal make-up.

The Body Shaping Diet matches your unique shape and hormonal make-up to the foods that will stimulate and re-balance your metabolism. This is what makes the Body Shaping Diet so effective, not only in the first few months, but for the rest of your life.

There will be no need to follow restrictive diets or feel hungry, weak and deprived, because by following the Body Shaping Diet you will feel satisfied, energetic and positively re-balanced. What's more you will lose weight where you want to, thus sculpting your physique into a more streamlined and balanced form.

ARE YOU READY TO MAKE A COMMITMENT TO THE BODY SHAPING DIET?

* Are you ready to lose weight efficiently?
* Are you ready to re-shape your body into a form that pleases you?
* Are you ready to tone and firm up and lose all your cellulite?
* Are you ready to feel feminine and more sexually alive?
* Are you ready to reduce your hormonal imbalances?
* Are you ready to feel more energetic, productive and increase your zest for life?
* Are you ready to improve your general health, well-being and boost your immune system?

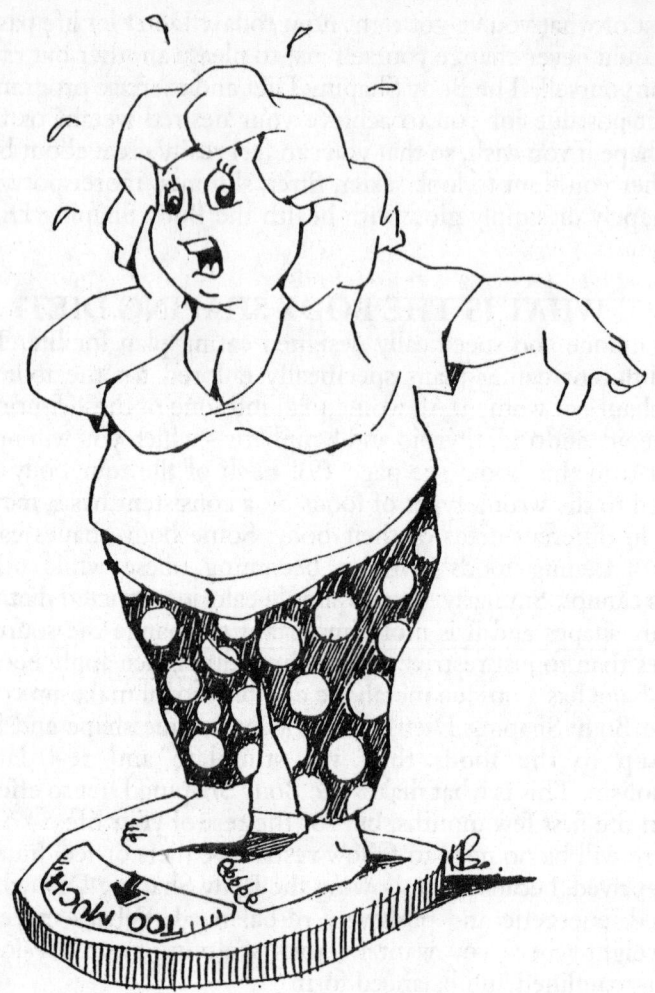

If your answers are Yes - you are ready to make the Body Shaping Diet commitment!

Congratulations on your decision to look and feel the best you possibly can. The Body Shaping Diet will streamline your body shape and give you the key to weight control, better health and feminine vitality.

WHY HASN'T SOMEBODY TOLD YOU THIS BEFORE?
The subject of 'women's hormones' or 'gynecological' endocrinology as it is called in medical terminology is a new speciality in medicine and doctors are only beginning to understand its powerful influence in our daily lives. The realisation that our body shape and weight are linked to

our dominant hormonal gland is also a new breakthrough with exciting and practical implications for women with excess weight.

For the first time ever we can now change our body shape and weight by re-balancing and fine-tuning the hormonal system through diet, nutritional supplements, exercise and, if necessary, hormone therapy.

The old-fashioned simplistic way of losing weight through restrictive dieting and heavy exercise may work for some, but not for all. Furthermore, in the long term 95 per cent of women who lose weight through restrictive low-calorie dieting will regain their undesirable weight. They will subject themselves to dangers such as extreme weight cycling, anaemia, loss of muscle tissue, increased risk of osteoporosis and mineral imbalances. In contrast, the Body Shaping Diet avoids unnecessary pain and hardship, does not put you at any risk and is guaranteed to work in the long-term.

For all body shapes we have a tailor-made programme of exercises to re-distribute fat and muscle tissue and help remove stubborn fat deposits and cellulite. These exercises complement the Body Shaping Diet (see page 221).

Investing our resources into our bodies is like investing our money. When and how we do it is crucial and in both endeavours it is vital to get the best professional advice. The designer of the Body Shaping Diet, Dr Sandra Cabot, has ensured that your valuable resources of time and effort will be rewarded by basing her program on many years of clinical experience and research.

HOW THE BODY SHAPING DIET WORKS ON THE CELLULAR LEVEL

To achieve weight loss and/or fat re-distribution, we need to stimulate the metabolism or chemical processes within our fat cells. The metabolic rate of our body is the rate at which the body cells convert food energy into physical (kinetic) energy. The metabolic rate of an individual appears to be the most important determinant of body weight. Those with a slow or sluggish metabolic rate gain weight most rapidly and lose weight most slowly. The Body Shaping Diet is designed to stimulate the metabolic rate of each fat cell bu providing it with the correct proportions of nutrients, vitamins, minerals, water and hormones. This enables you not only to burn food calories at a faster rate, but facilitates the breakdown and/or re-distribution of stubborn inactive fat deposits. Thus, weight loss and body re-shaping becomes quicker, easier and if you stick to the Body Shaping Diet, long lasting.

Let's don the cap of a scientist for a moment and take a look at a fat cell under the microscope–see diagram 2. As you can see the raw materials required for the chemical processes within each fat cell are:

hormones, vitamins, minerals, oxygen, fats, carbohydrates and protein. If these raw materials are out of balance - say, for example, too many sex hormones, not enough vitamins and minerals, not enough oxygen and too much saturated fat - then the inner chemical processes of the fat cells do not occur efficiently and we have a reduction in the metabolic rate. If this continues, weight gain is sure to result with accumulations of sluggish, underactive fat cells appearing. Here we have the microscopic genesis of cellulite and layers and ridges of unsightly fat.

You can now understand why it is vital to follow an eating plan that works on each individual fat cell if you are really going to change your body weight and shape in an efficient and lasting way. The Body Shaping Diet will do this by providing each fat cell with the correct proportions of vitamins, minerals, fats, protein, carbohydrates and water.

Diagram 2

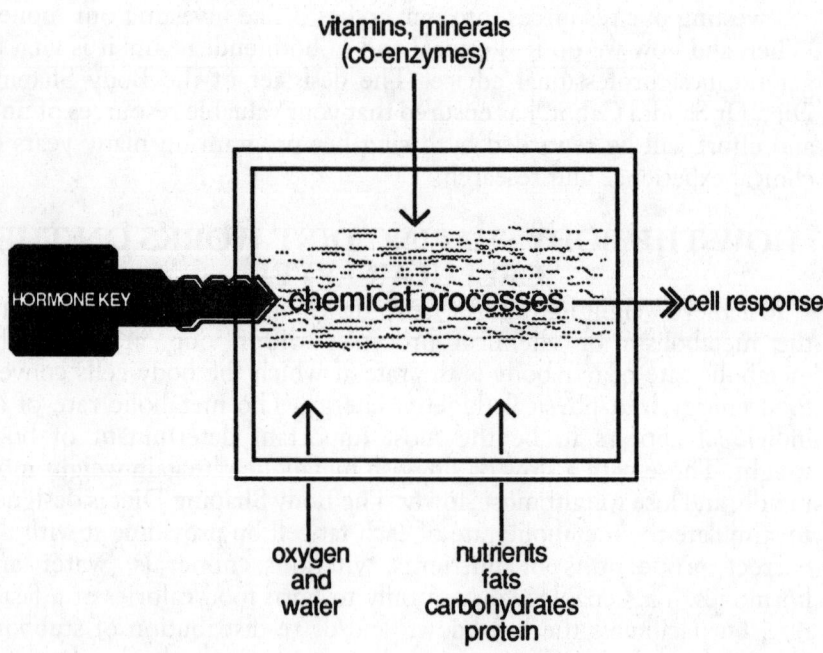

A FAT CELL

In addition, the Body Shaping Diet will re-balance the cellular metabolism specifically for each of the four different body shapes - android, gynaeoid, thyroid and lymphatic. The metabolism of the fat cells is different in each of the four body shapes and each shape requires a unique balance of vitamins, minerals, fats, proteins and carbohydrates.

When the correct balance of these nutrients for each body shape is supplied in the diet, we not only stimulate the metabolism of each fat cell, but also achieve a re-balancing of the hormonal (endocrine) system. It is this latter effect that promotes the re-distribution of body fat so that the body shape can begin to change in a way that pleases us - that is, more streamlined and balanced from head to toe.

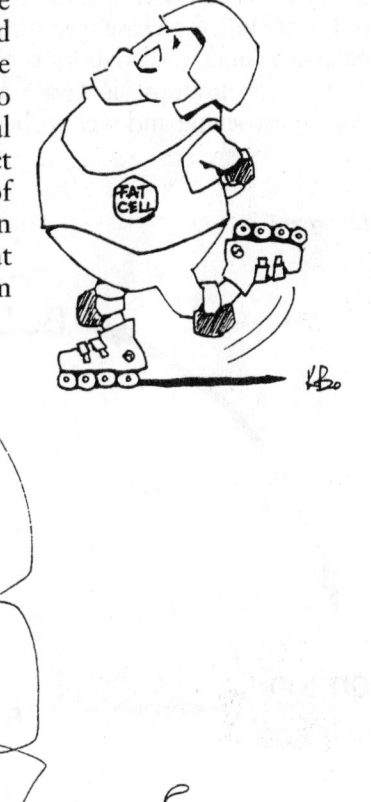

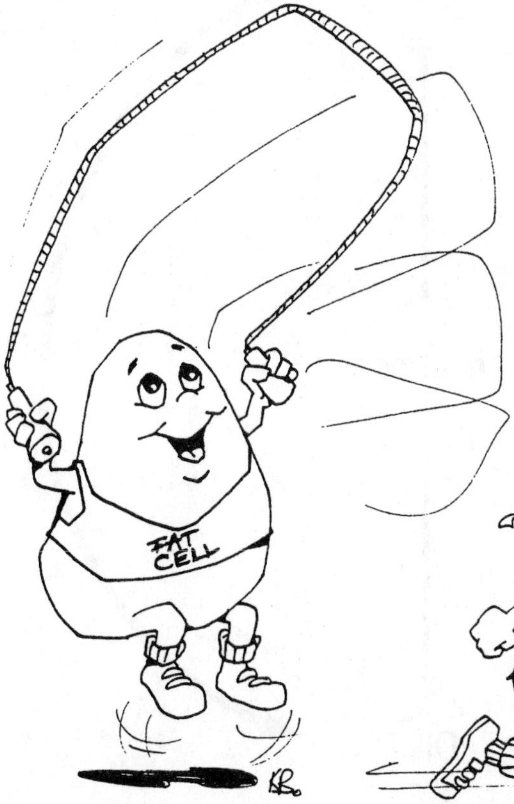

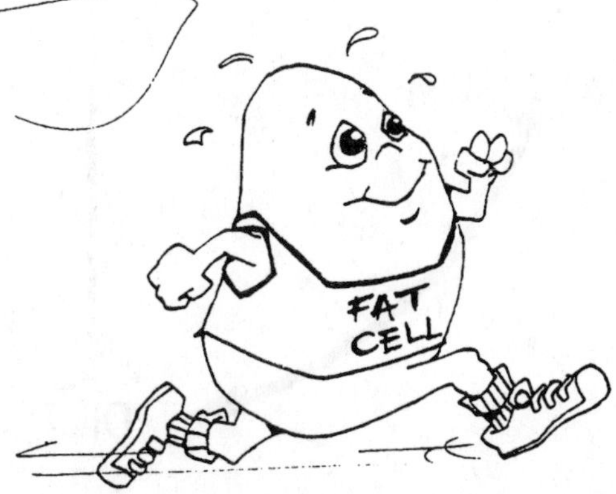

It is the missing links between **BODY SHAPE—DIET—HORMO-NAL BALANCE,** that are so vital and have previously prevented women from changing their body shape. Of course, exercise is important too, and you can see from diagram 3 how all these factors influence each other. Standard calorie restricted diets are limited - they only enable you to lose weight temporarily, but don't produce an overall balancing and re-distribution of body fat. The Body Shaping Diet and exercise programme is a safe and effective permanent way to change your body shape and weight because it fills in the missing links.

Diagram 3

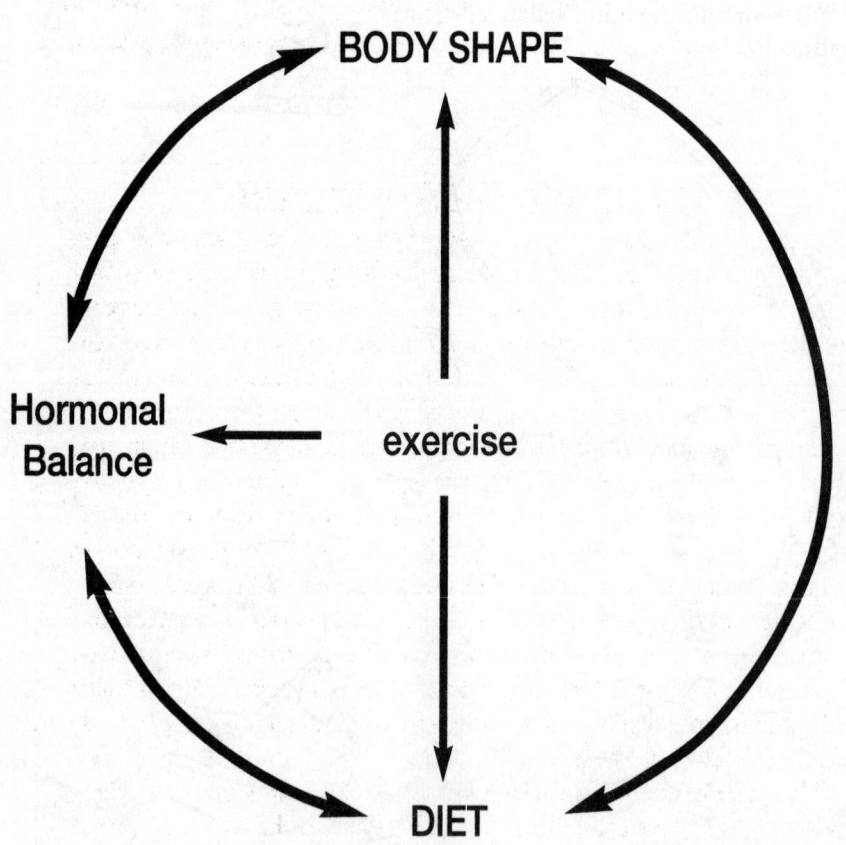

CHAPTER ONE

HOW TO RECOGNISE YOUR BODY SHAPE

To fit yourself into one of the four female body shapes look at the diagrams beginning on page 20 and compare yourself to these, full frontal and sideways, while standing naked in front of the mirror. Choose the body shape that most closely resembles your own. You can also visit the web site www.weightcontroldoctor.com and do an interactive questionnaire which will determine your body type.

THE ANDROID SHAPE

This shape is characterised by a strong, thickset skeletal frame with large shoulders, a large rib cage and muscular limbs. The neck, chest and abdomen are rather thick and the pelvis is small so that android women are relatively straight up and down. They lack feminine curves and have muscular buttocks and powerful muscular thighs. The pelvis and buttocks do not curve outwards very much below a rather thick waist.

Android women are somewhat masculine in shape and often make good athletes in sports requiring strength and staying power, such as body building, swimming and long distance running. They may be told that they resemble their fathers or brothers and yet these women are very attractive and glow with health. The bones in their limbs, hands and feet are large and they have more muscle mass and less fat tissue than most women unless they become overweight. If weight gain occurs, fat is deposited in the upper part of the body—above the pelvis. This produces a thickening of the neck, trunk, waist and abdomen and gives rise to the term 'apple-shaped' obesity.

The android woman may also have skin problems such as excess facial and body hair (hirsutism), acne and hair loss from the scalp in the male pattern of hair loss. These things are the result of her higher levels of male hormones.

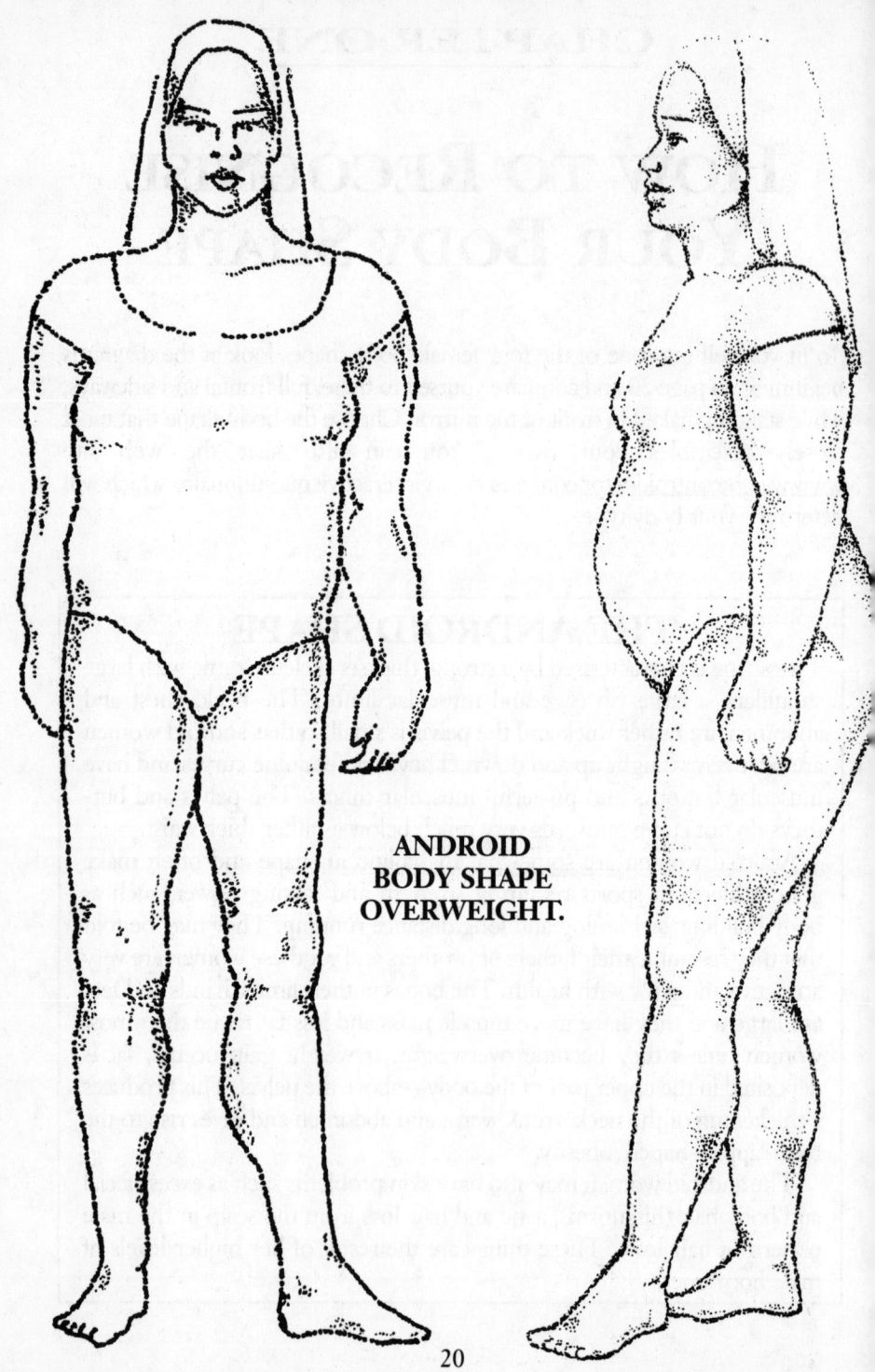

**ANDROID
BODY SHAPE
OVERWEIGHT.**

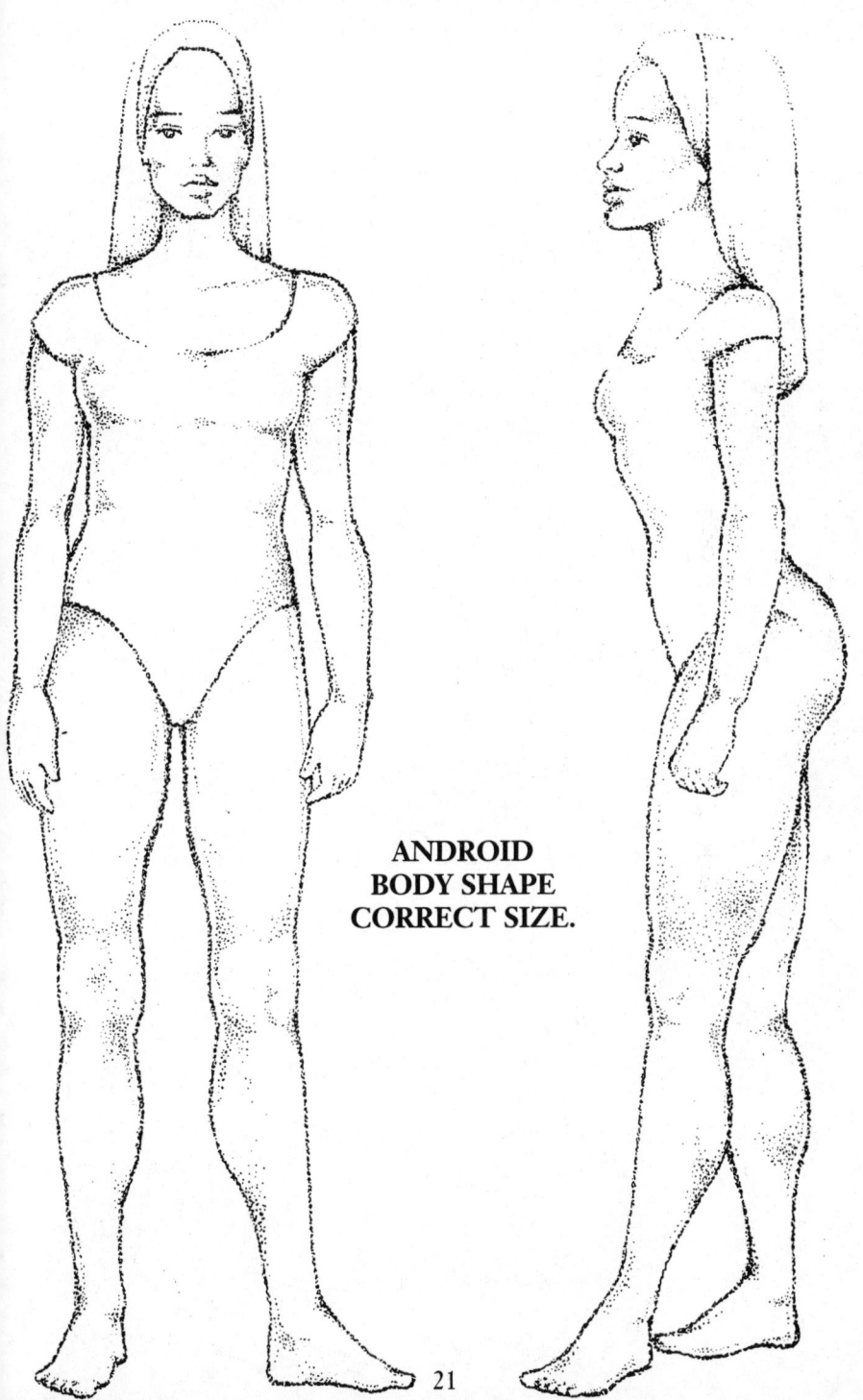

**ANDROID
BODY SHAPE
CORRECT SIZE.**

THE GYNAEOID SHAPE

This shape is characterised by a pear shape, with the body flaring outwards towards the hips and thighs. The buttocks are curved and rounded and the thighs are curved outwards laterally and may touch together on the inside or medial aspect. The bottom has a tendency to droop downwards (posterially) over the back of the thighs. The waist is tapered and smaller than the hips giving a feminine appearance. The breasts are variably sized and may be small to large. The shoulders are small to moderate in size. Typical measurements for a gynaeoid woman are 39", 29", 43".

The bones of the arms and legs are feminine with tapered, fine forearms, wrists, shins and ankles. Even if obesity occurs, the forearms and shins remain relatively fine and slim with fat tissue accumulating firstly on the thighs, buttocks, breasts and later over the lower abdomen in front of the pubic bones. The bones of the pelvic cavity are wide, thus giving rise to the term 'good childbearing hips'. Gynaeoid women tend to produce more estrogen and are "estrogen dominant". The majority of women fit into the gynaeoid shape.

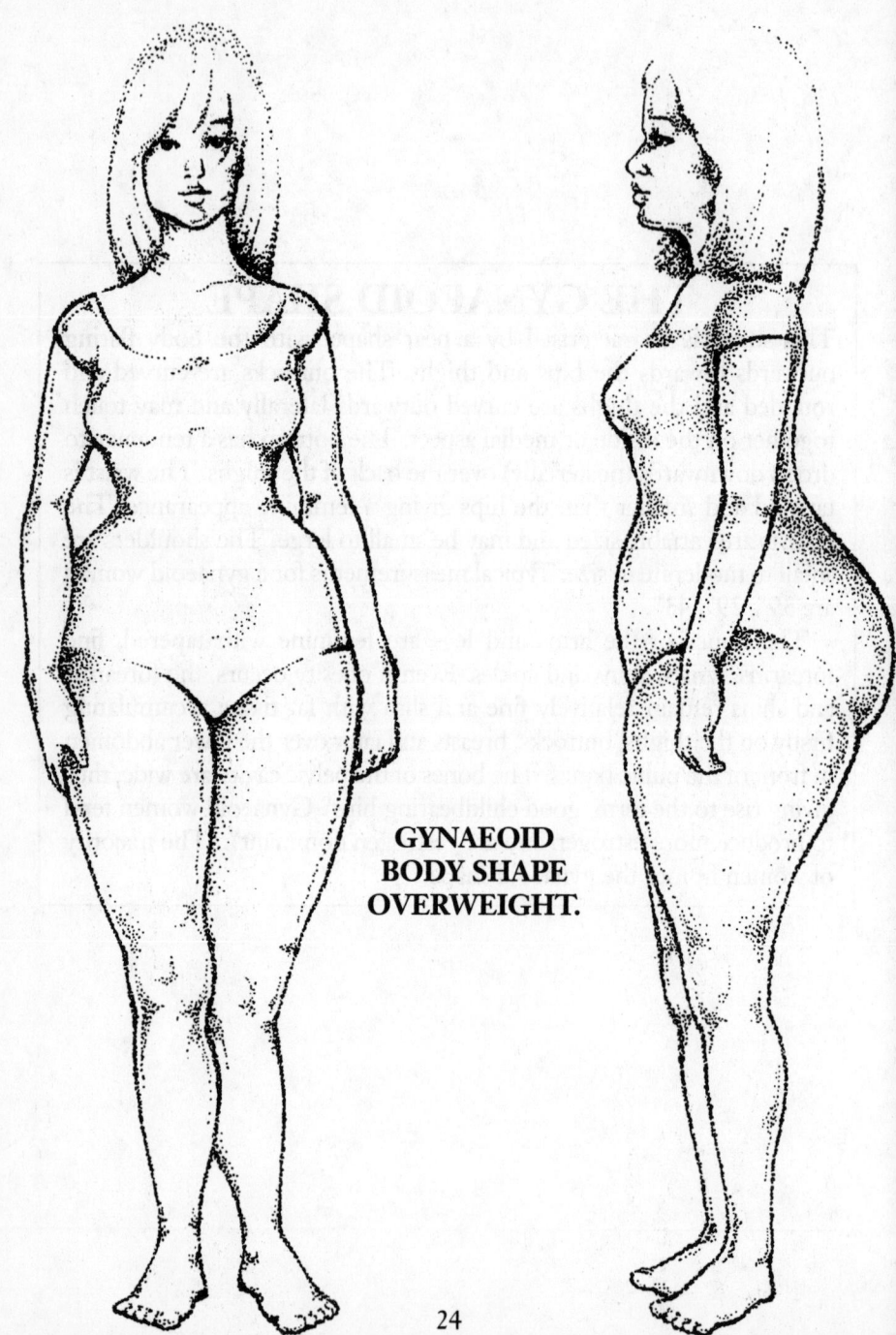

**GYNAEOID
BODY SHAPE
OVERWEIGHT.**

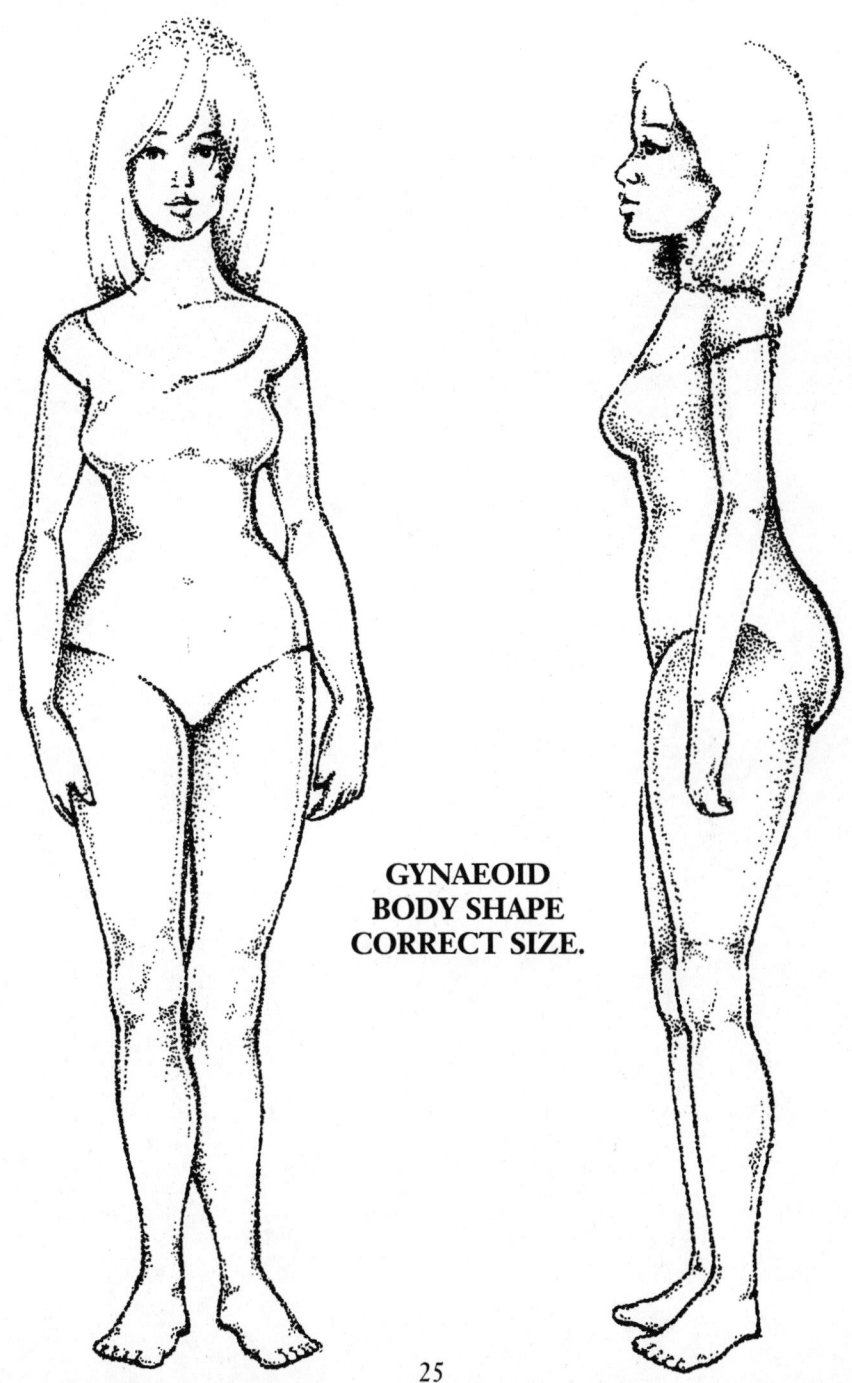

**GYNAEOID
BODY SHAPE
CORRECT SIZE.**

THE LYMPHATIC SHAPE

The lymphatic-shaped woman is characterised by a generalised thickening and puffiness of the body. This is due to the fact that she retains water easily especially in her limbs which gives her thick arms and legs with a straight up and down look along their length. The ankles and wrists are thick and puffy in appearance. The shoulders, breasts and rib cage are small to average in size and the abdomen protrudes in front. The trunk, like the limbs, is relatively straight up and down with a thick waist and moderate outward curves on the buttocks and pelvic area.

The bones of the skeleton and the muscles are average in size and their shape is not clearly defined as they are covered by a thickish layer of fat and fluid. In other words it is difficult to see their bone structure and they are definitely not the 'bony type' which we find amongst thyroid-shaped women.

The thick straight up and down look comes from the accumulation of fluid and fat in the tissues under the skin (subcutaneous layer) which is evenly distributed over the bone and muscle structures. If a lymphatic woman becomes obese her fat will be distributed all over her body, in the legs, feet, arms, hands, buttocks, abdomen, trunk, neck and face. Lymphatic women have often been 'chubby' since childhood and resemble a 'cupid' or 'cuddly baby doll' and most find that they gain weight easily.

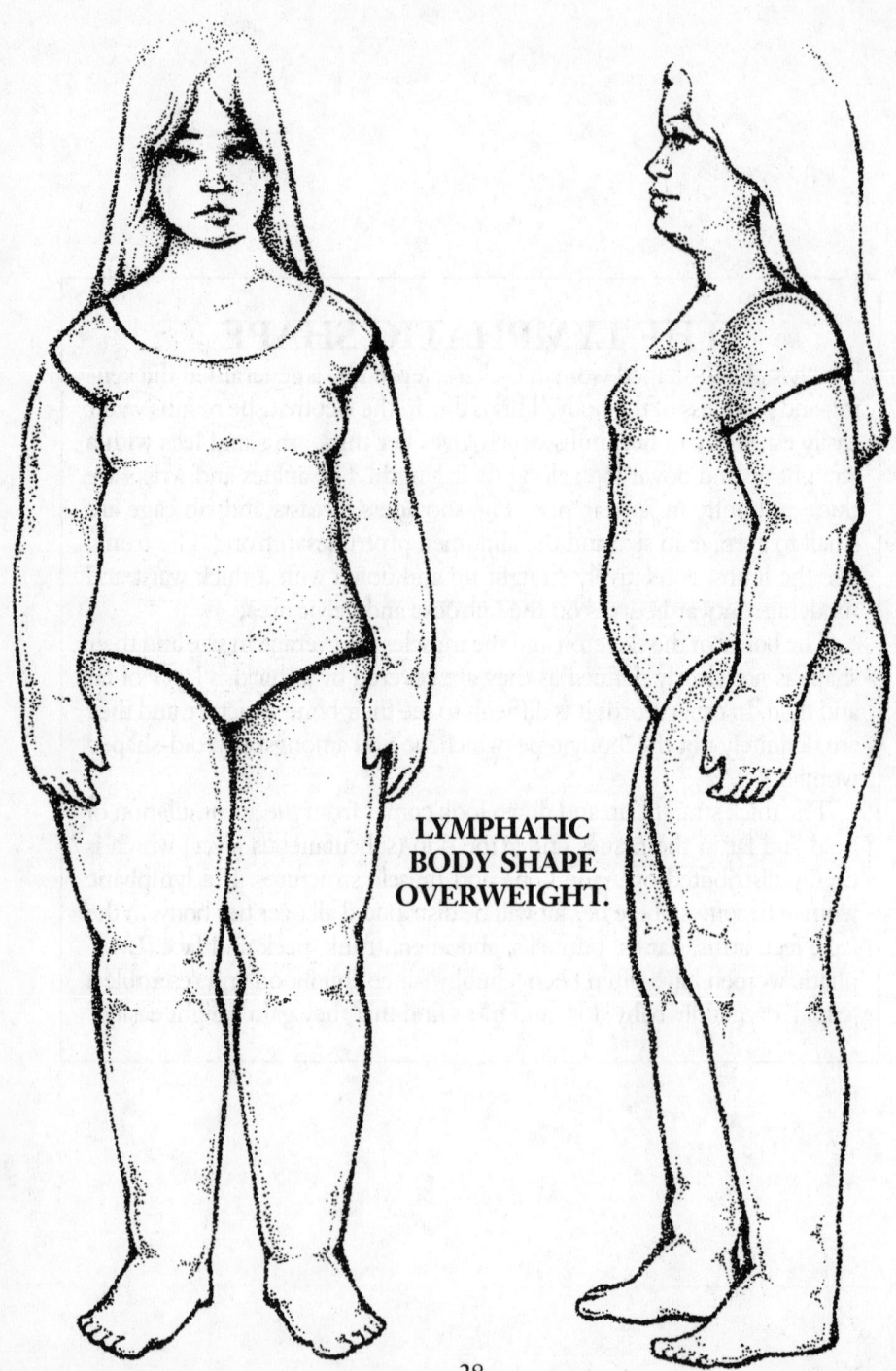

**LYMPHATIC
BODY SHAPE
OVERWEIGHT.**

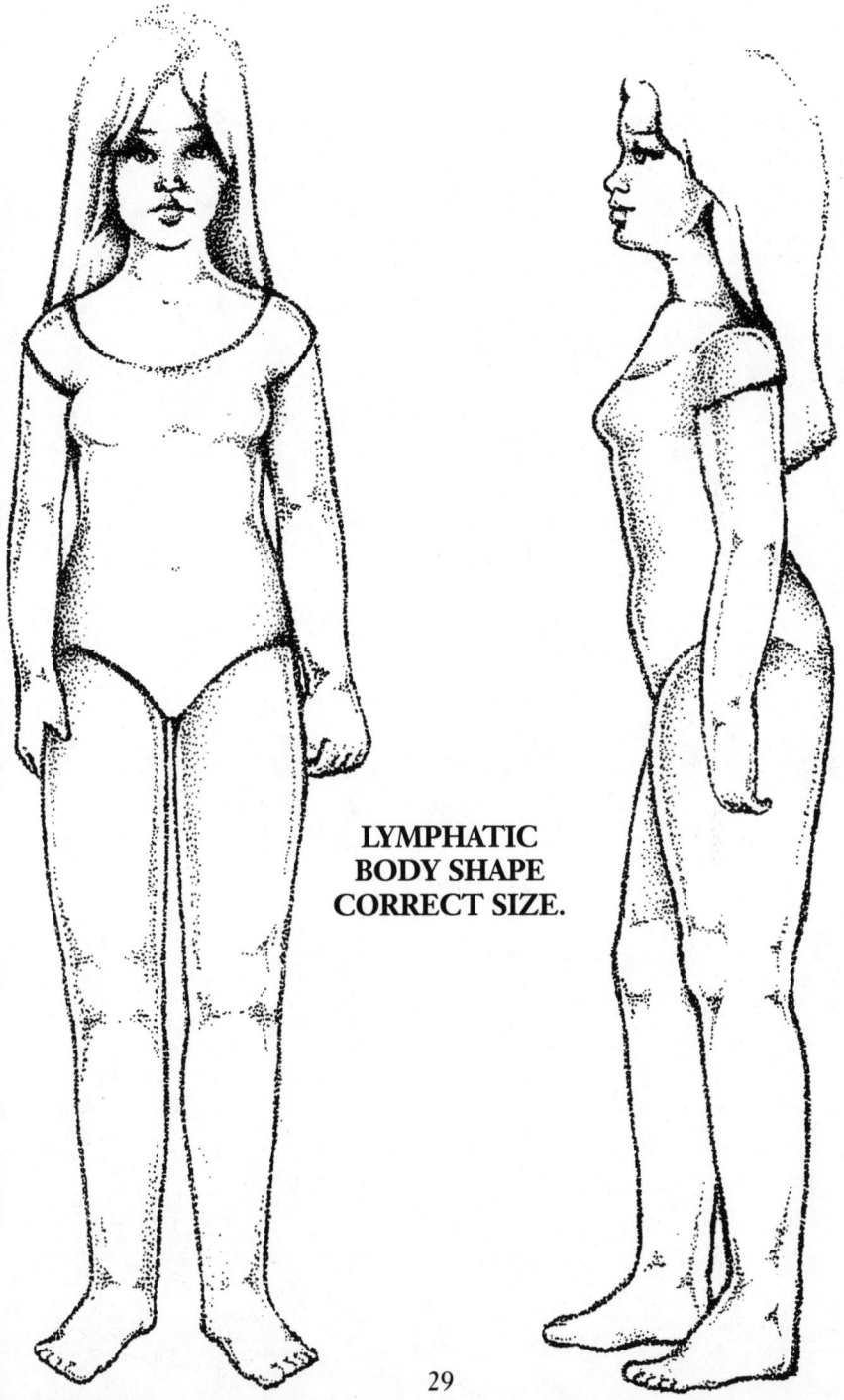

**LYMPHATIC
BODY SHAPE
CORRECT SIZE.**

THE THYROID SHAPE

The thyroid woman is characterised by a narrow streamlined shape with long limbs and fine bones. The long arms and legs produce a 'thoroughbred racehorse look'. The breasts tend to be smallish although they may be moderate in size. Thyroid-shaped women are often tall, but even if they are not, they give the impression of being tall because of their long fine limbs. They have a 'slender' figure with a narrow waist and generally only small curves on the buttocks and thighs. They move gracefully and may be athletes, especially sprinters or basketball players, dancers or one of today's models. Twiggy and Jerry Hall are the epitome of the thyroid shape.

Their fingers and toes are long and fine to match their limbs and their necks are long and tend to be narrow. They could be described as 'willowy' meaning willow tree like and may have a fragile look about them. Their bones are small to average in size and the bone structure is clearly defined beneath a thin layer of subcutaneous fat. They are often bony in appearance with their ribs and bony protuberances (knobs) around their joints being very evident.

If weight gain occurs, fat is first deposited around the abdomen and upper thighs with the upper part of the body remaining slim.

**THYROID
BODY SHAPE
OVERWEIGHT.**

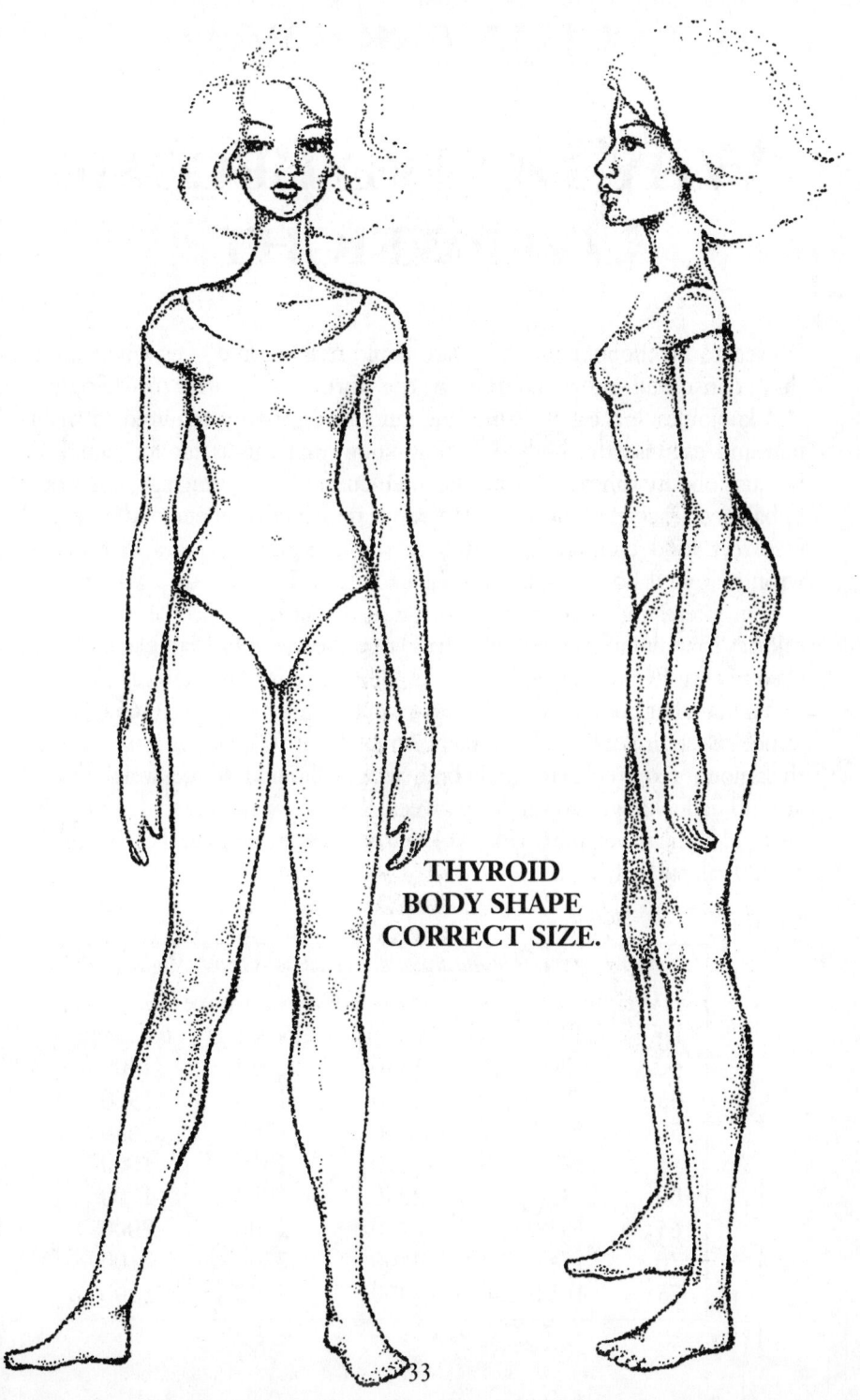

THYROID BODY SHAPE CORRECT SIZE.

CHAPTER TWO

WHY DO WE BECOME OVERWEIGHT?

It used to be thought that a person could not become overweight unless they consumed more energy in the form of calories or kilojoules (4.2 kilojoules = 1 calorie) than the amount of energy required to maintain and exercise the body. We now know that this is far too simplistic because obesity can occur from the interaction of increasing age, emotional imbalance, incorrect hormone therapy, underactive metabolic rate and incorrect food combining as well as the consumption of a diet that is wrong for your body shape. This will all be explained shortly.

It is interesting to note from diagram 4 that small people need fewer calories to maintain their weight than larger people. For example, a woman aged twenty-five years weighing 40 kg (88 lb) needs only 1550 calories daily to maintain her body weight whereas a woman weighing 75 kg (165 lb) at the same age requires 2400 calories daily. An intake of 500 calories a day less than the amount required to maintain body weight should lead to a weight loss of around half a kilogram (1 lb) every week. Thus, you can see that a forty-five year old woman weighing 65 kg (143 lb) could lose one pound each week on a 1600 calorie daily diet.

Diagram 4 (lb=pound)

Calories required for maintenance of various body weights				
Weight		Calorie Intake		
kg	lbs	25 years	45 years	65 years
40	88	1550	1450	1400
45	99	1700	1600	1550
50	110	1800	1700	1650
55	121	1950	1850	1800
60	132	2050	1950	1900
65	143	2200	2100	2000
70	154	2300	2200	2100
75	165	2400	2300	2200

However, this simple balancing equation does not work for every woman! I have seen countless women who have rigorously matched the calories they consumed to the number of calories they used up for body maintenance and exercise, only to find that they slowly continue to gain weight. They usually came to see me in a very confused and frustrated state and were often suffering from depression. Later I was able to reveal to them the reasons why they could not lose weight by explaining the factors affecting the metabolic rate of their fat cells (diagram 2 on page 16).

Let us review these reasons and how they thwart our well-meaning attempts to lose weight by calorie restriction alone.

1. Increasing Age

As we advance in years, the chemical processes or metabolic rate of our cells slows down. Thus, we gradually begin to burn calories at a slower rate. Many pre-menopausal and menopausal women will relate to this as they begin to develop a middle-age spread around the abdomen.

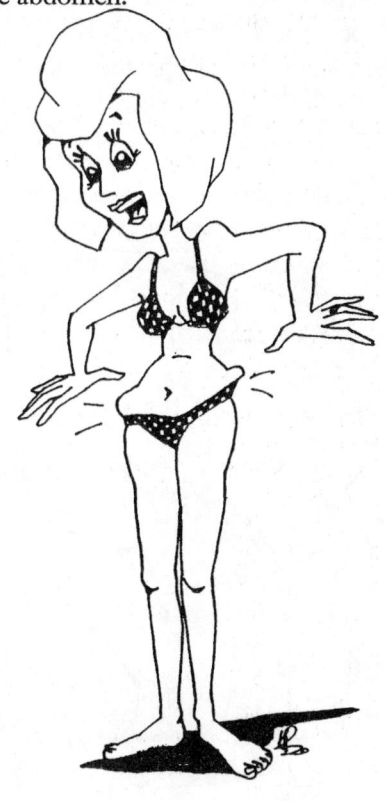

This annoying tendency can be avoided by regular exercise (at least forty minutes daily) and by reducing the amount of saturated fats in the diet. Foods that are high in saturated fats and which must be avoided are: full-cream dairy products, fatty and processed meats, processed and takeaway foods and fried foods. Older women should replace these undesirable foods with grains, cereals, legumes, lean meats, seafood, fresh fruit and vegetables.

Furthermore, as we age our cells become more dehydrated, in other words they have a reduced water content. This causes a slower elimination of toxins and waste products from our cells which results in sluggish chemical processes within the cells. To offset this poor metabolism, older women should increase their intake of water to 35 to 70 ounces daily, and reduce their intake of sugary drinks and alcohol.

They will also benefit from the natural supplement called METABOCEL, which increases the metabolic rate and makes it much easier to lose weight (see page 247).

By following these simple steps you will avoid becoming fat, matronly or middle-aged in appearance. Start well before the menopause so that it does not catch you unawares.

2. Emotional Hunger

Many women are so-called 'comfort eaters'. In other words, they may not really be hungry for food but they eat or drink when they feel depressed, helpless, powerless, rejected, lonely, ugly, poor, angry, frustrated or bored. In such cases, they are feeding their minds and souls with calories which, of course, only act as a temporary distraction or 'painkiller'. Some women are afraid of their sexuality or of the opposite sex and subconsciously feel that by appearing overweight and undesirable, they will not have to deal with these aspects of womanhood. As this method of self-defence is operating in the deeper subconscious mind, they may not be aware of the true nature of these fears, but only know that they somehow feel better when surrounded by a 'suit of armour' in the form of a thick layer of fat. Such women may have been hurt or rejected in love affairs, sexually abused or be victims of incest.

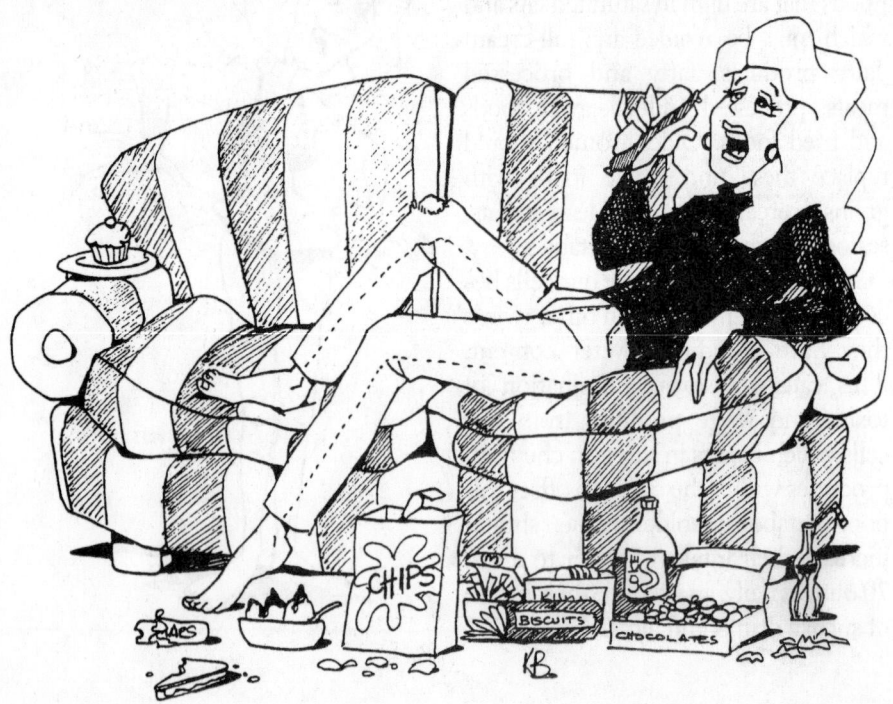

Thus, obesity can be a symptom of emotional lack or imbalance and this should be looked for, especially if obesity is associated with anxiety, depression or mood disorders.

These problems can be overcome by working on your self-esteem and self-image. Very few of us are perfect and we can go a long way by accepting ourselves and making the best of our positive attributes. I see many women who do not appreciate the value of their own worth and need to increase self-esteem, self-confidence and assertiveness before dieting can become easy and effective.

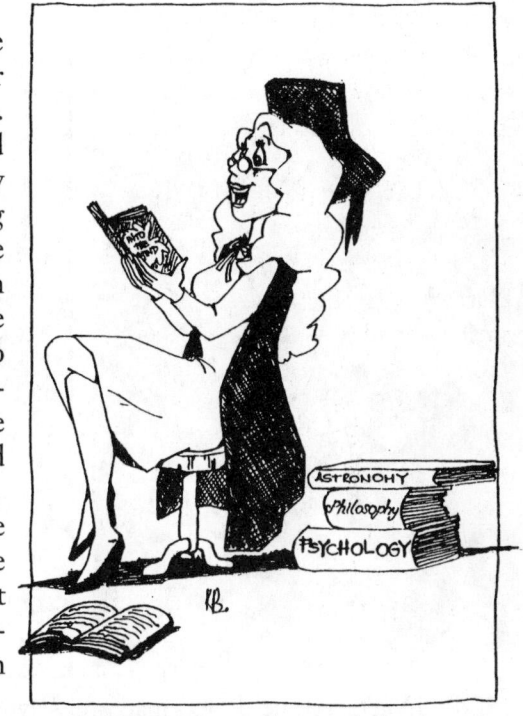

Strategies that can fill the void of emotional hunger are many and varied and are not the subject of this book. However, there are a few worth mentioning:

a) Undertake counselling or psychotherapy to understand the reasons for your behaviour. Read books on psychology, psychiatry and self-discovery. You can buy these or borrow them from a library.

b) Learn and practise meditation as it takes you back to the source of your being and enables you to know and love your inner self.

c) Be daring and do something you have always wanted to do but put on hold for a trillion reasons. Starting early and doing it little by little is better than delaying it for too long. Live your life as an exclamation, not as an explanation!

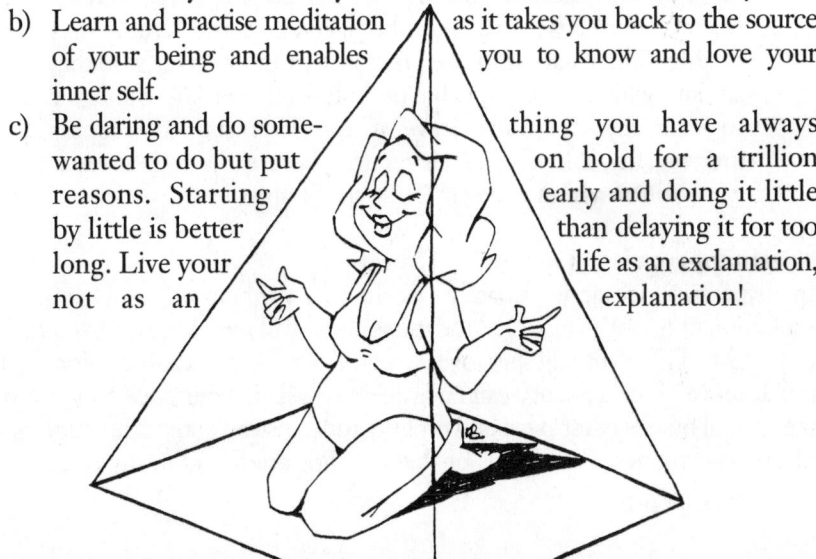

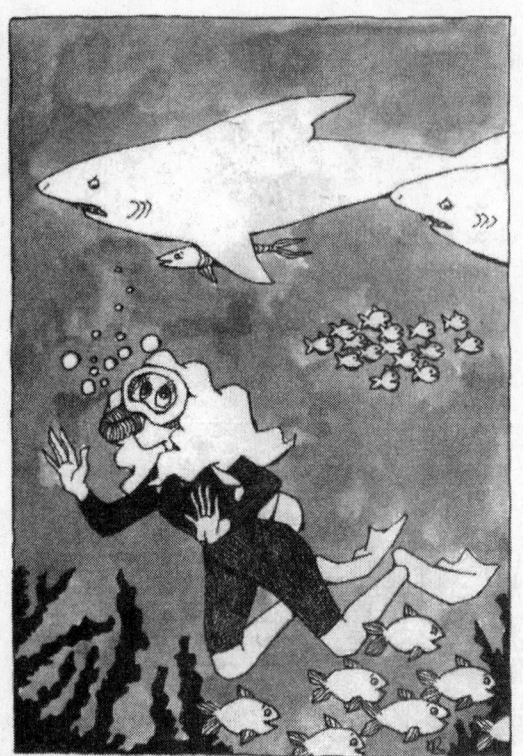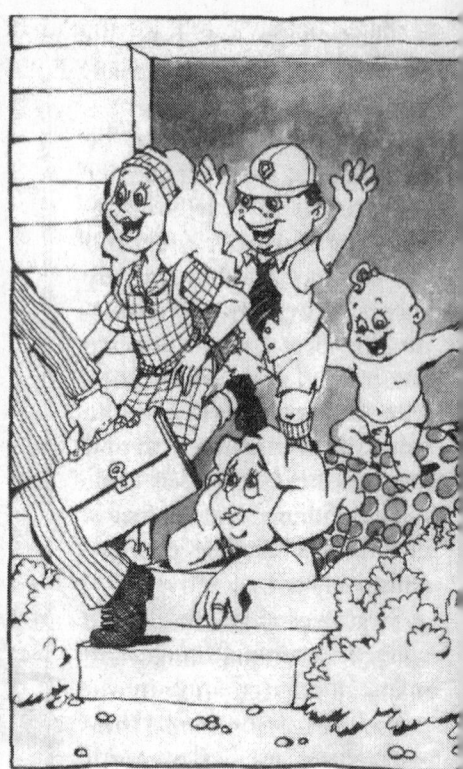

d) Don't become a 'doormat' and slave to your partner, husband and children—tell them you need time to develop your own mind, body and soul. Take time for exercise, buying health foods and developing your intellect and creative talents. Many wives and mothers reach menopause and find themselves in the 'empty nest syndrome'. They have forgotten themselves and wonder who they really are and what they are capable of. You will never know unless you try, so take my tip, don't leave it too late, start developing your individuality, talents and desires way before the menopause; otherwise you may find yourself eating to fill up your empty nest.

3. Inappropriate Hormone Therapy

In my experience approximately one in two women who start hormone replacement therapy (HRT) at the menopause will gain a significant amount of weight. This is usually just over 2 kg (4–5 lb) but it can occasionally be much more. This tendency can be avoided by asking your doctor to give you the natural brands of estrogen and progesterone, instead of the synthetic brands of these hormones. Full details of these brands are found in my book titled

Menopause—HRT and its Natural Alternatives, published by the Women's Health Advisory Service. Quite a few menopausal ladies find that they need to reduce their dosage of hormone replacement therapy or failing that, take their hormone replacement therapy in the form of the estrogen patch or cream, instead of tablets, to avoid gaining weight.

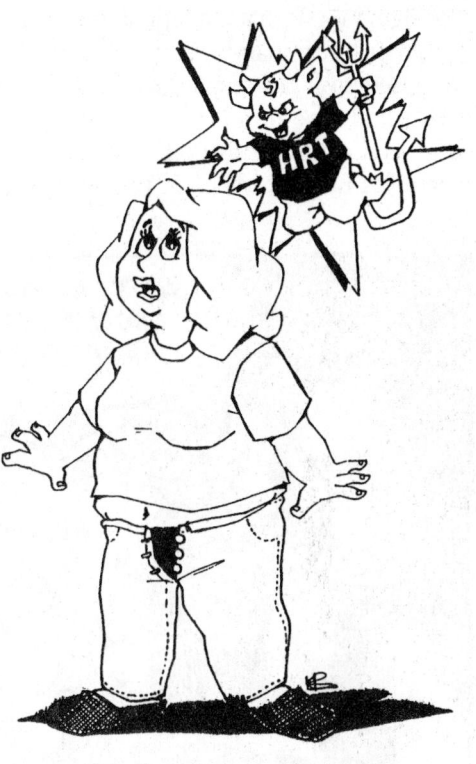

Generally speaking, heavier women require a smaller dose of hormone replacement therapy than lightweight or thin women. They may need to take a smaller amount of progesterone, either by breaking the tablet in half or quarters or by taking it for a shorter time in each calendar month. Natural progesterone is less likely to put on weight than are synthetic brands of progesterone—namely, Primolut and Provera.

The estrogen patch is available under several different brands and comes in three strengths—100, 50 and 25.

The smaller doses in the weaker estrogen patches, for example, the 25 and 50 strength, or the estrogen creams are most unlikely to cause weight gain. Generally speaking, it is possible, by juggling and/or reducing the doses of estrogen and progesterone in your hormone replacement therapy, to avoid any significant weight gain.

If, despite all these measures, hormone replacement therapy still causes unwanted weight gain, you may decide to give it away altogether, but check with your doctor first as you may be losing the great advantages that estrogen replacement therapy has for your skeleton and blood vessels. If after all consideration you decide to give hormone replacement therapy away, I suggest you consume a diet that is high in calcium, vitamin D and natural food sources of estrogen. Natural plant estrogens can be found in many foods such as green beans and soya beans and for full details of foods high in natural plant estrogens, see page 74.

To find foods that are high in calcium see our Calcium Table on page 196.

Other hormonal drugs that can cause unwanted weight gain are the oral contraceptive pill (especially high-dose formulas) that contain synthetic masculine type progesterones. Ask your doctor for one of the newer low dose oral contraceptive pills containing friendly, feminine progesterones—examples of these types of progesterones are gestodene and desogesterol.

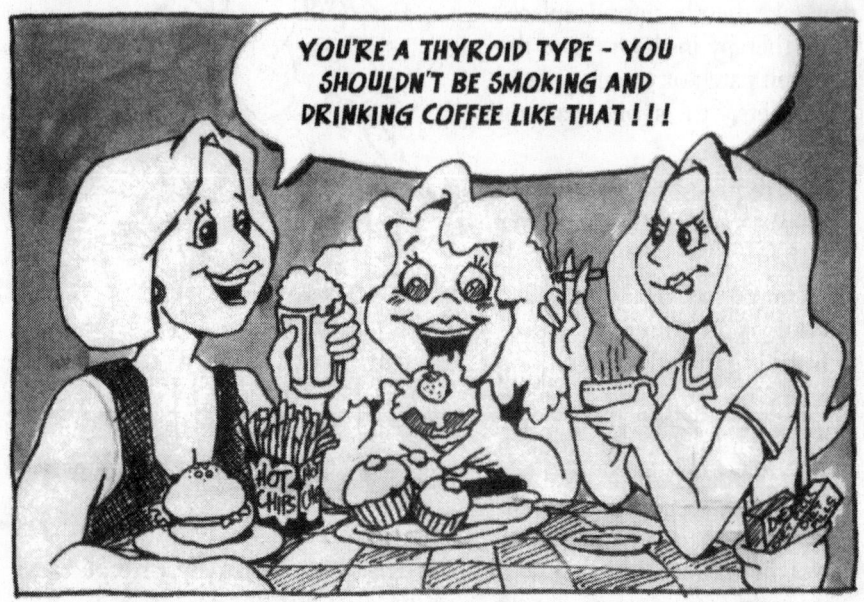

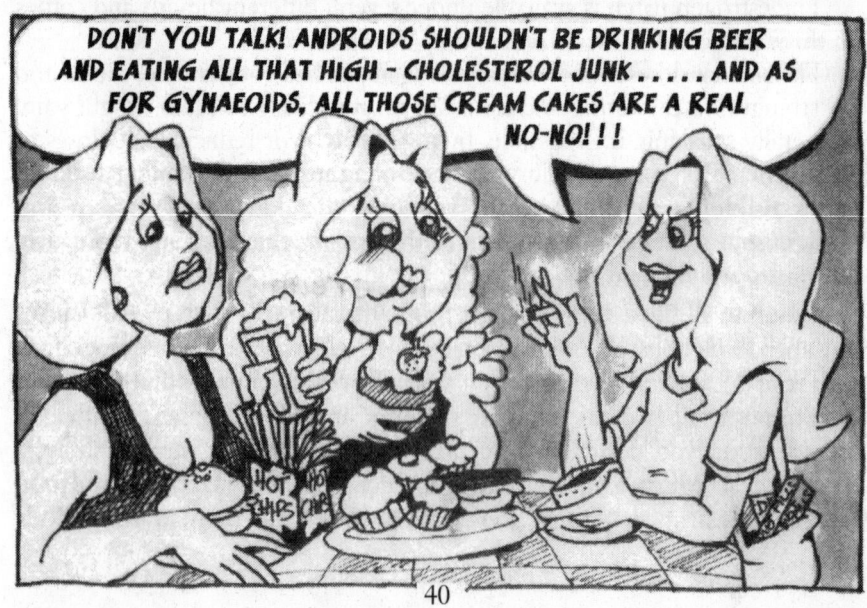

These have far less tendency to stack on extra weight.

Women taking anabolic steroids for competitive sport and athletics gain both muscle and fat, whereas the hormone cortisone used in a variety of medical diseases causes an accumulation of fat in the face and abdomen. This can be offset by exercise and usually disappears once the medication is discontinued.

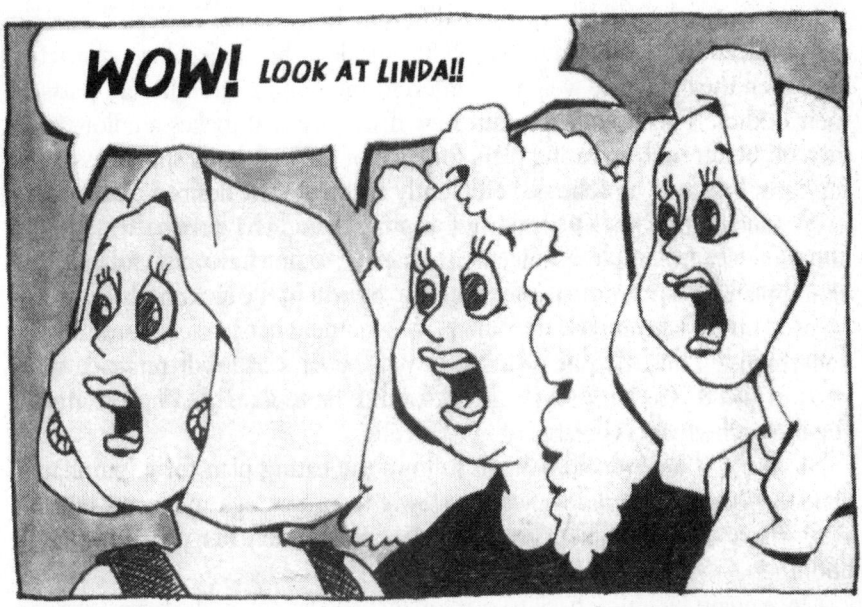

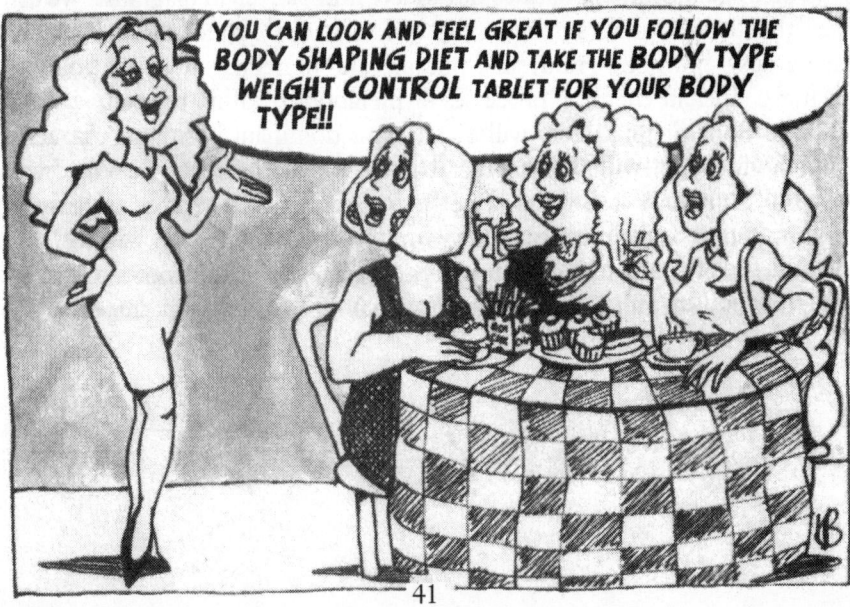

By going back to diagram 2, you can see that hormones act as powerful keys on our cells and greatly influence the chemical processes within the cells. Thus the type and amount of any hormonal replacement or drugs that you are taking, especially on a long-term basis, must be carefully chosen and reviewed regularly by your doctor.

4. The Wrong Diet For Your Body Shape

If four women, each one being a different body shape or type—namely gynaeoid, android, thyroid or lymphatic—follow the same calorie restricted diet, then they will lose weight at different rates and from different parts of their bodies. This is an important new discovery that makes a tailor-made diet, or, better said, an eating plan, for each of the four body shapes essential if weight loss is to be achieved efficiently and from the desired places.

No one diet will work properly for all women and I have seen this time and time again. For example, if a gynaeoid-shaped woman follows the eating plan for a thyroid-shaped woman, she will lose weight in the face and breasts, but not from the areas she has unwanted fat—namely her buttocks and thighs. Thus, despite restricting her calories she will retain a large bottom and thighs because she is not eating the types of foods to stimulate the inner chemical processes of her fat cells.

Similarly, if an android woman follows the eating plan for a lymphatic-shaped woman she will lose weight slowly from her legs and arms, but not from the areas where she is prone to obesity—namely her neck, trunk and abdomen.

Once again by going back to our lonely little fat cell in diagram 2 we can see that it is vital to surround the cell with the correct balance of raw materials—hormones, nutrients, vitamins and minerals—if we are going to achieve efficient chemical processes or metabolism within the cell.

The Body Shaping Diet will match your dominant hormonal character and body shape with the correct balance of fat, protein, carbohydrate, vitamins, minerals and water. The Body Shaping Diet recipes are easy to follow and we explain the way they work on your metabolism. We will also include specific nutritional, naturopathic and herbal supplements to stimulate metabolism and aid weight loss for each of the four body shapes.

CHAPTER THREE

HOW IS YOUR PRESENT WEIGHT?

Simply by looking in the mirror it can be difficult to judge just how overweight or underweight you are. Perhaps you would prefer not to know! For those of us who would like to know, the table below shows us if we fall into the desirable or normal weight range for our height and frame size.

Desirable Weight age 25 years and over

Height		Small frame		Medium frame		Large frame	
cm	ft	kgs	lbs	kgs	lbs	kgs	lbs
142	4'8"	42-44	92-98	44-49	96-107	47-54	104-119
145	4'9"	43-46	94-101	44-50	98-110	48-55	106-122
147	4'10"	44-47	96-104	46-51	101-113	49-57	109-125
150	4'11"	45-49	99-107	47-53	104-116	51-58	112-128
152	5'0"	46-50	102-110	49-54	107-119	52-59	115-131
155	5'1"	48-51	105-113	50-55	110-122	54-60	118-132
157	5'2"	49-53	108-116	51-57	113-126	55-63	121-138
160	5'3"	50-54	111-119	53-59	116-130	57-64	125-142
163	5'4"	52-56	114-123	54-61	120-135	59-66	129-146
165	5'5"	54-58	118-127	56-63	124-139	60-68	133-150
168	5'6"	55-59	121-131	58-65	128-143	63-70	139-154
170	5'7"	57-61	126-135	60-67	132-147	64-72	141-158
173	5'8"	59-64	130-140	62-68	136-151	66-74	145-163
175	5'9"	61-65	134-144	64-70	140-155	68-76	149-168
178	5'10"	63-67	138-148	65-72	144-159	69-78	153-173

Note: For ages between 18 and 25 years, subtract half a kilogram or one pound for each year under 25 years of age.

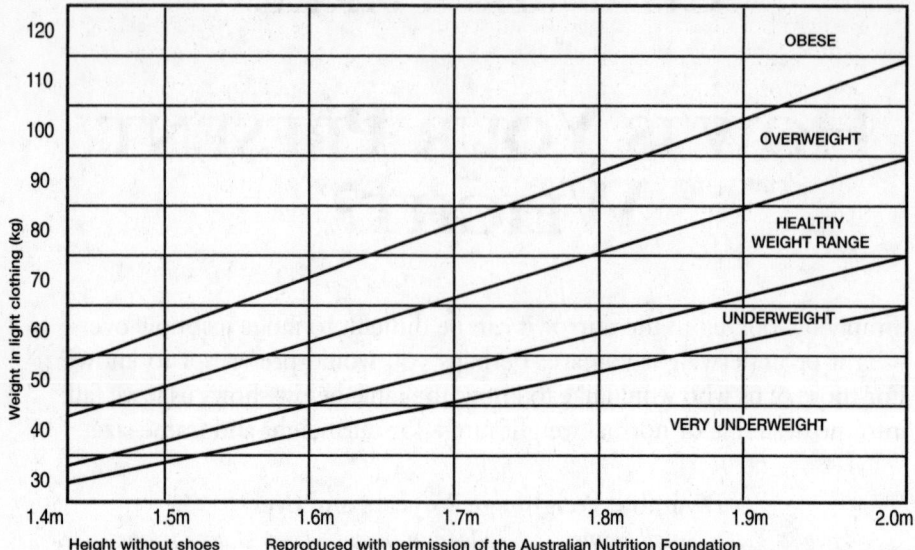

WEIGHT FOR HEIGHT (Use this chart to plot weight and progress)

Diagram 5   *(one kilogram = 2.2 pounds, one metre = 3.28 feet)*

Another more graphic way of illustrating your weight can be done by plotting your weight (along the vertical axis), alongside your height (along the horizontal axis) on the weight for height graph.

If you fall into the obese range of the graph you may be subject to the following medical risks:

1. High blood pressure and cardiovascular disease.
2. Diabetes.
3. Respiratory problems.
4. Gall stones.
5. Complicated pregnancies.
6. Arthritis.
7. Increased risk of cancer of the breast, uterus, gall bladder and bowel.
8. Hormonal and gynecological disorders such as fibroids and heavy painful periods. Obesity will cause a women to make more estrogen in her fatty tissues and this stimulates the growth of fibroids and may worsen endometriosis and increase menstrual blood flow and pain. As android women get fatter their level of the male hormone testosterone increases, which will increase the tendency to facial hair, greasy skin and acne. Weight loss will correct these hormonal imbalances and consequently improve gynecological and skin problems.

9. Sleep apnea, which is the medical term for failure to breathe during sleep. This affects the hypothalamus and reduces oxygen supply to the cells, which reduces the metabolic rate and makes it much harder for you to lose weight. Sleep apnea in obese persons can have severe effects causing a reduction in testosterone production in males and a big reduction in the amount of growth hormone produced by the pituitary gland. These effects may increase the rate at which the body ages.

10. A shorter life span and higher risk of death.

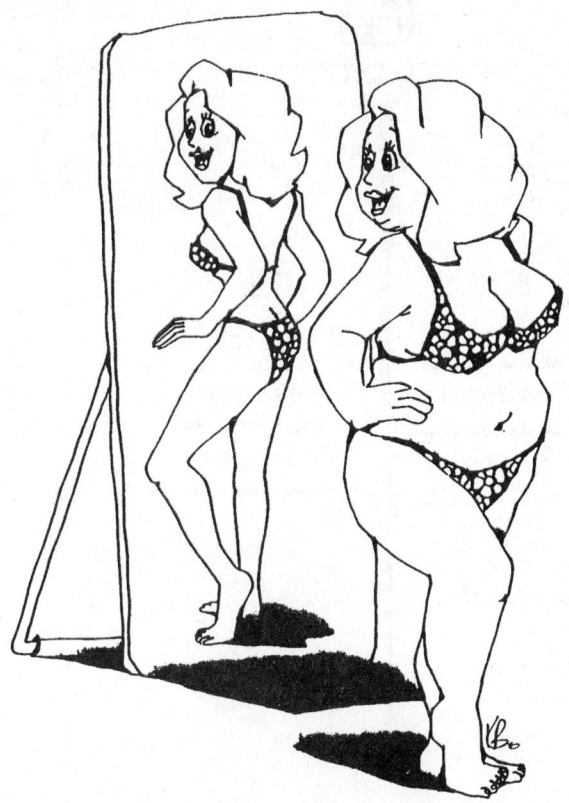

Never lose sight of your goal!

If you fall into the overweight range on the graph, you will also be subject to the above ten medical risks but with less susceptibility than those in the obese range.

If you fall into the very underweight range on the graph, you should try to gain weight by increasing your consumption of calories and protein foods to increase fat and muscle tissues. Try to eat more bread, cereals, grains, nuts, whole-meal cakes, honey, fruits, eggs, chicken, seafoods and lean meats.

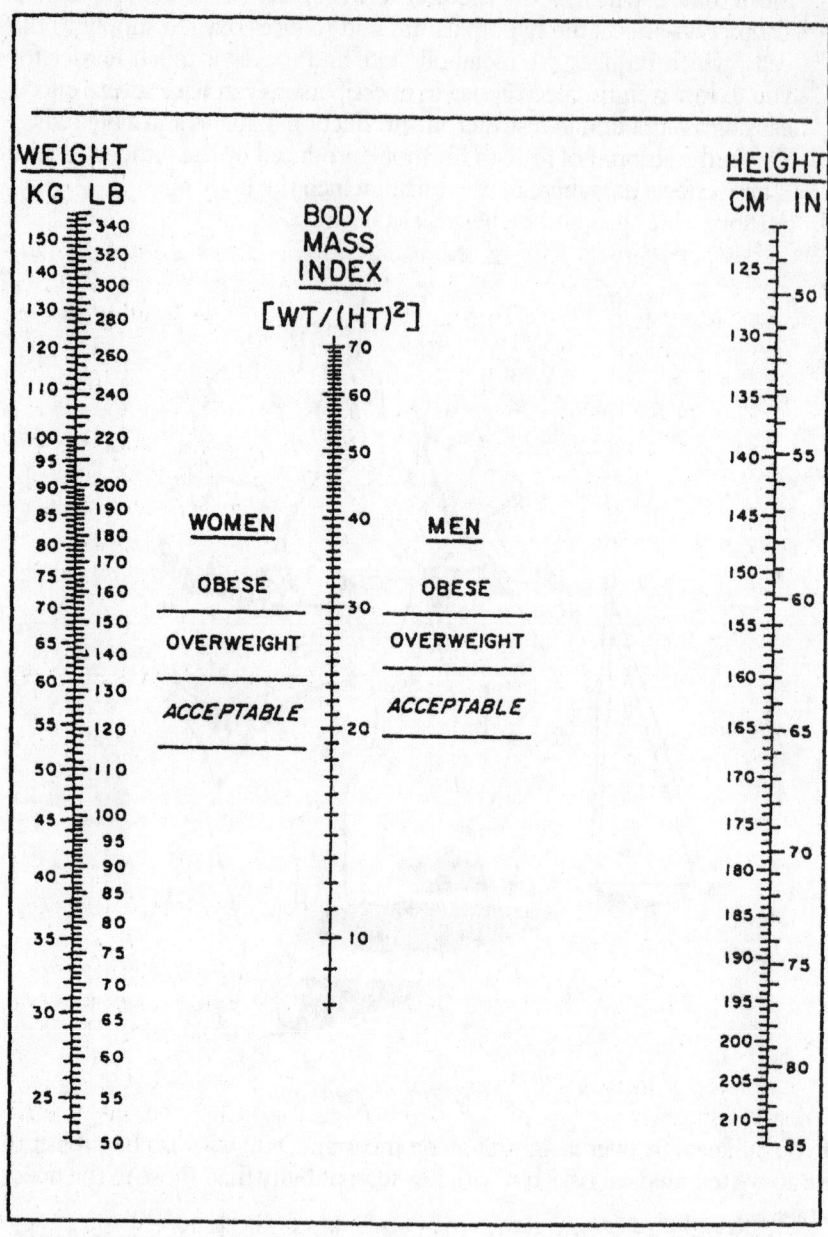

Diagram 6

If you remain very underweight, you will be at an increased risk of the following disorders:

1. Low levels of estrogen with an associated higher risk of osteoporosis and cardiovascular disease.
2. Reduced fertility.
3. Complicated pregnancies.

By understanding your weight-for-height ratio, your body type and the factors that determine your metabolic rate, you are now in a powerful position to change the things that prevent you from achieving the healthy weight range depicted on our graph.

BODY MASS INDEX (BMI)

The most scientific way of looking at your weight is a ratio or equation known as the body mass index (BMI). For those not good at maths don't tune out, as it is really very simple! You can calculate your body mass index by dividing your weight (in kilograms) by the square of your height (in metres) i.e.:

$$\text{BMI} = \frac{\text{WEIGHT (KILOGRAMS)}}{\text{HEIGHT X HEIGHT (METRES)}}$$

For example, if you weigh 75 kilograms and are 1.69 metres (169 centimetres) tall then your

$$\text{BMI} = \frac{75 \text{ KILOGRAMS}}{1.69 \times 1.69 \text{ METRES}}$$

$$= \frac{75}{2.856}$$

Your **BMI** = 26.26 (an electronic calculator will make this easier to work out).

If you don't like equations, you can easily work out your BMI from the scale on page 46. To use it place a ruler between your weight (undressed) and your height (without shoes). Then read your BMI on the middle scale.

• If you are a woman you should aim to keep your BMI between 19 and 25 depending upon your build; for men BMI should fall in the range of 20 to 26. By keeping your BMI in these ranges you will enjoy better general health.

• Overweight is considered between the upper limit of normal body mass index (25 for women) and a body mass index of 29.

• Obesity is defined as a body mass index greater than 29.

• Anorexia nervosa (see page 230) is associated with a body mass index of less than 17.

When weighing yourself choose the **same time** of the day, wearing no clothes. Weight can vary by 2½-4½ pounds over one day, due to fluid retention, constipation, a full bladder, exercise, hormonal changes, time of the menstrual cycle and other factors. Thus, weighing yourself once or twice a week is sufficient, less frustrating and less prone to small errors.

THE BODY SHAPING EATING PLAN STRATEGY

The body shaping eating plan consists of two simple steps:

1) STEP ONE

TO LOSE WEIGHT. This is desirable if your body mass index is over 25. You can use the body shaping diet menus, found between pages 92 and 118 to bring your weight back down into the ideal body mass index range of 19 to 25.

2) STEP TWO

TO MAINTAIN IDEAL BODY WEIGHT. Once you have achieved a weight and body shape that pleases you it is important that you do not discard the Body Shaping Diet. At this stage, ideally, your weight will fall into the body mass index range of 19 to 25. To maintain your desired weight and figure follow the BSD menus found between pages 119 and 137 and practise the body shaping exercises beginning on page 221.

CHAPTER FOUR

THE ANDROID-SHAPED WOMAN

The classical android-shaped woman is rather square shaped with a solid big-boned frame giving her a powerful and athletic appearance. Her dominant gland is the adrenal gland, of which there are two situated on top of each kidney. These two small fleshy glands produce the powerful hormones cortisone and adrenalin as well as a variety of male hormones (androgens). The android woman will have a tendency to over-produce male hormones, particularly if she becomes obese. These male hormones will make her look more masculine and may stimulate the growth of facial and body hair, greasy skin and acne.

The powerful adrenal hormones make her energetic and strong with good staying power when others around her need a coffee break or sugar fix. Android-shaped women are usually not sugarholics or 'sweet tooths', but instead crave foods high in cholesterol and salt that act to stimulate their dominant adrenal glands to pump out more steroid hormones, such as cortisone and androgens. These hormones are anabolic, meaning that they promote an increase in body muscle and fat which accumulates around the jowls, neck, shoulders, upper arms, trunk and abdomen. This further exaggerates the tendency towards a masculine appearance.

If android women become overweight, the excess fat is deposited in the upper half of the body, i.e. above the hips and we call this upper-level body obesity, which contrasts with the lower-level body obesity typical of gynaeoid-shaped women. Android or upper-level body obesity is more dangerous for health than lower-level body obesity as it is associated with a higher level of the medical complications of obesity such as cardiovascular disease, high blood pressure, high cholesterol and diabetes. These things may shorten life span.

Thus, it is important to encourage android-shaped women to maintain their body weight within the normal range for their height or more specifically to maintain their body mass index (see page 46) in the normal range of 19–25 kg/m^2.

Body fat is a significant source of production of the sex hormones estrogen and androgens (male hormones). As the amount of fat in the body increases, so will the amount of estrogen and androgens produced in the fat increase. Conversely, weight loss and a reduction in body fat is associated with a lowering in levels of estrogen and androgens. Thus, it is easy to understand how hormonal imbalances can be corrected by weight normalisation.

The Body Shaping Diet for android-shaped women (see page 91) is scientifically designed to help weight loss and hormonal imbalance in two ways:

1. It is low in cholesterol, saturated fat and salt, which will reduce the excessive production of androgens from the adrenal glands.
2. It promotes weight loss in the upper part of the body and abdomen and this further lowers body androgen levels.

All women produce both male and female hormones in their ovaries, adrenal glands and fat. Indeed, women chemically convert male hormones into female hormones and if a woman does not produce male hormones, she will make less estrogen. If the levels of androgens are excessive compared to the levels of the female hormone estrogen, the body shape becomes more masculine and acne may occur. What we are aiming to achieve with the Body Shaping Diet is a re-balancing of the levels of female and male hormones (androgens). Reducing male hormone levels and upper-body fat causes the appearance and body physique to become more feminine.

POLYCYSTIC OVARY SYNDROME

At this point it is worthwhile mentioning a rather common hormonal disorder that is more likely to occur in android-shaped women, especially if they become overweight. This is called the polycystic ovary syndrome and in this disorder the ovary looks different to a normal ovary (see diagram 7). In a normal ovary, the eggs or follicles are distributed evenly throughout the ovary whereas in the polycystic ovary, follicles varying in size from 2–8 millimetres are lined up around the edge of the ovary. The polycystic ovary does not function in an ideal way and usually produces excessive amounts of male hormones and does not produce a regular supply of fertile eggs. Thus the menstrual cycle is usually irregular and most commonly menstrual bleeding is infrequent, occurring only two or three times per year.

Obesity may trigger the polycystic ovary syndrome and will cause it to be more pronounced. In obese women the large deposits of fat produce excessive male hormones which act on the polycystic ovary and stimulate it to produce even more male hormones.

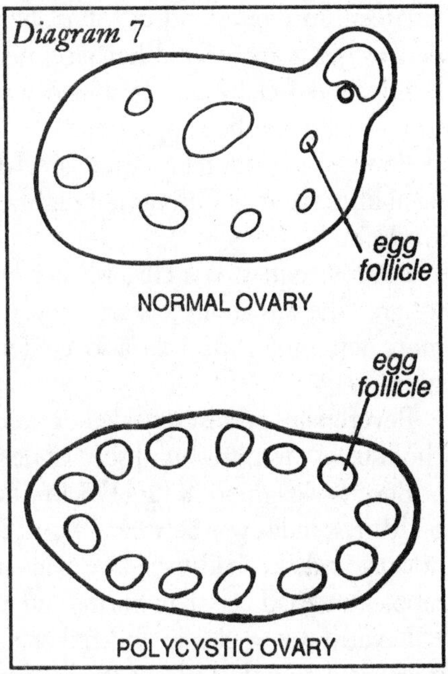

Thus, in obese android women with polycystic ovary syndrome we have three sources of production of excessive male hormones—the fat, the adrenal glands and the ovaries. Little wonder that many of these women complain of acne and excess facial and body hair. If the level of male hormones becomes very high, loss of scalp hair may occur with the hair thinning in the frontal and temporal areas of the scalp.

Mild cases of polycystic ovary syndrome can often be corrected simply by losing excess weight and women with polycystic ovaries should keep their body mass index around 21 kilogram/m². Ideal weight equals height² (metres²) x 21 (reference: *Women's Hormone Problems*, Dr John Eden, First Edition 1991). Thus if you are 170 cm (5'8") in height your ideal body weight = 1.7 metres x 1.7 metres x 21 = 60.69, or approximately 61 kg (134 pounds).

Diagram 7

egg follicle

NORMAL OVARY

egg follicle

POLYCYSTIC OVARY

Once ideal weight is achieved, regular menstrual bleeding often resumes and male hormone levels reduce with a resultant decrease in acne and facial hair. More severe or resistant cases of polycystic ovary syndrome will require the use of specific hormone therapy designed to block the effect of the excess male hormones and produce a regular menstrual cycle. This tailor-made hormone therapy will cure acne and greatly reduce facial hair. Hormones that may need to be used for this are cyproterone acetate, estrogen and natural progesterone.

In android-shaped women with very high levels of male hormones, weight loss can be easier and more effective if the excess of male hormones is corrected first, which can be done with hormone therapy.

BEVERLY'S CASE HISTORY

Beverly was a very mature woman for her age of twenty-five and exuded an air of relaxed confidence and power which enabled her to successfully run a large furniture factory. She had been struggling with excess body and facial hair for seven years ever since she had started to gain weight at the age of eighteen. In typical android style, her weight gain was mostly in the upper part of her body around her face, neck, chest and abdomen. Her excessive weight and facial hair, combined with her android shape, gave Beverly a somewhat masculine appearance.

Beverly's periods had started late, when she was seventeen, and had always been infrequent so I thought it highly likely that she had the polycystic ovary syndrome.

Beverly requested a cure for her excess hairiness and assistance in losing weight. She was about to start a new relationship and wanted to look and feel more feminine. She was also contemplating having children in her late twenties.

Beverly's blood test revealed excessive levels of male hormones and raised cholesterol. An ultrasound scan of her pelvic area showed polycystic ovaries.

Beverly weighed 78 kg (173 lb), her height was 165 cm (5'5") and her body mass index was between 28 and 29. Her blood pressure was higher than normal and she had excessive hair around her chin, upper lip, navel and nipples and had very hairy arms and legs

Beverly was a classic android-shaped woman with the added hormone imbalance of polycystic ovary syndrome. She craved fatty and salty foods such as pizza, salami, ham and fish and chips. These foods were stimulating her adrenal glands to produce excessive amounts of male hormones, which had gradually increased her body hair and weight over the last seven years. Beverly was utterly amazed to learn that her beloved fish and chips could be increasing her body hair and masculinity, as she had not realised that a high-fat diet could cause a hormone imbalance. She had thought that she simply took after her father and that she was destined for shaving cream and the razor blade.

Beverly was started on the Body Shaping Diet for android-shaped women (see page 92). The menus in this eating plan contain foods that are high in estrogenic substances which would have a feminising effect upon her physique. See page 74 for a complete list of foods high in natural estrogens. The Body Shaping Diet for android women contains protein that comes mainly from non-animal sources such as grains, cereals, nuts, seeds, legumes and fish. These protein sources are high in fiber and low in saturated fat and salt and they do not stimulate the adrenal glands to produce anabolic hormones. Only small servings of organic chicken, lean red meats and low-fat dairy products are allowed in the Body Shaping Diet for android women. Battery hens should be avoided as they may be fed anabolic hormones to make them grow quickly, only free range organic chicken should be eaten.

Liver-friendly foods such as garlic, onion, chives, dandelion, watercress, beetroot and carrots are included as they act as tonics for the liver. An active and healthy liver is required in android-shaped women because the liver breaks down and inactivates the steroid hormones which tend to be present in excessive amounts.

Beverly applied her enormous enthusiasm and willpower to following the Body Shaping Diet (see page 91 for android women) and was pleased to see results after only two months. She had lost 8 kg (17.6 pounds) in weight and had slimmed down over her upper body. Her blood pressure was now normal and her cholesterol levels were down by two points.

Beverly was anxious to have a regular menstrual period and reduce her facial hair so I recommended that she start a tailor-made oral contraceptive pill containing two different hormones. This contained the female hormone estrogen and an anti-male hormone Androcur (Cyproterone Acetate), which would block the effect of her excessive male hormones upon the hair follicles. Androcur is a potent anti-male hormone and has been proven to cure acne and greatly reduce excess facial and body hair. It is a slow-acting hormone and I explained to Beverly that Androcur would take a full twelve months to fully exert its effect in controlling body hair.

Well, after twelve months one could hardly recognise Beverly as the same person who had originally presented to me looking overweight, hairy and masculine. She now weighed 57 kg, (125 lb) which for a height of 165 cm (5'5") put her body mass index at 21, which was ideal for a woman with polycystic ovary syndrome.

She no longer looked obese and solidly square in shape and indeed looked slim and decidedly feminine. Her facial features looked finer as did her neck and muscular limbs. Her previously large pendulous breasts and protruding abdomen were no longer obvious as she had lost large amounts of weight from these areas.

Beverly was very happy in her relationship and said that for the first time in many years she now felt like a woman and loved looking feminine. She assured me that she intended to remain that way and would stick to the Body Shaping Diet and exercise programme for the rest of her life.

FREIDA'S CASE HISTORY

Freida came from a Germanic background and had inherited the stocky android frame of her grandmother. She had worked hard with her husband on their large property growing grains and raising cattle for thirty years and had recently moved to the city. She was forty-nine and just beginning the menopause and wanted to avoid the middle-age spread. With this aim in mind she avoided sweets and cakes but continued to enjoy a diet high in meats, cheese and salty foods. Freida was having trouble in maintaining her body weight and had started accumulating fat around her neck, upper arms and abdomen which was not surprising due to her adoption of a more sedentary lifestyle and her high-fat diet. She complained to me that her appearance was becoming more masculine and that she noticed increasing amounts of hair growing on her face.

On examination, Freida weighed 168 pounds which for her height of 5'3", put her body mass index between 29 and 30. Her blood pressure was slightly raised and blood tests revealed very low levels of the female hormone estrogen, in keeping with her menopausal state, and normal levels of male hormones. Freida's increasing facial hair was due to the fact that now she was menopausal, her hormonal balance had changed and she had relatively more male hormones than female hormones. Her ovaries were no longer producing significant amounts of hormones and her supplies of male hormones were coming from her increasing fat supplies and her adrenal glands.

Thus, I explained to Freida that if we were to reduce her levels of male hormones we would need to change her diet, so that her body fat reduced and her adrenal glands were not over stimulated. The perfect diet for this aim, and the one that also matched her body shape, was the Body Shaping Diet for android women. This diet was a slight cultural shock for Freida, whose central European family had always thought that red meats, eggs, dairy products and salty foods were the foundation of a strong, healthy body.

Still, we agreed it is never too late to change one's way of thinking and Freida decided to try the recipes and menus in the Body Shaping Diet for android women. She began eating far more raw fruits and vegetables, grains, legumes, seeds, nuts and fish than she had ever done, and gradually began to taste the more subtle flavours of food, as her meals were no longer seasoned with salt. Initially, she really missed her fried foods especially her Vienna schnitzel, but as she began to notice her body shape changing her satisfaction and pleasure made it easier to resist these high-fat foods.

Six months after her first visit, Freida was no longer craving salt and fried foods and told me that her favourite food was now vegetable and mixed bean soup. She felt that she had formed an entirely new set of taste buds on her tongue. Freida had lost 27½ pounds and now weighed 140 pounds (63.5 kg) which for her height of 5'3" (160 cm) put her body mass index just under 25. She looked far more feminine as her neck and shoulders had slimmed down and her abdomen was now flat and muscular. This was due to the combination of the Body Shaping Diet for android-shaped women and the body shaping exercise programme which had also brought her blood pressure back to normal and increased her fitness.

Freida felt so good about her new self that she now wanted to start hormone replacement therapy to eliminate her facial hair and stop hot flushes. I started her on a combination of natural estrogen and a small dose of the anti-male hormone Androcur which would stop the male hormones from stimulating her facial hair follicles.

Twelve months later Freida looked fit, trim and feminine and her facial hair was greatly diminished. She was content to stay on the Body Shaping Diet for her shape indefinitely, with a few special treats thrown in at birthdays and holiday times.

MAGGIE'S CASE HISTORY

Maggie had travelled a long distance from one of Australia's country towns to consult me about her rapid gain in weight of 44 pounds (20 kg) in just over two years. She had gone from 134 pounds (61 kg) to 178 pounds (81 kg), which for her body height of 5'3" (157.5 cm) gave her a body mass index of just over 31.

She was confused, depressed and totally bewildered because she had gained this weight despite the fact that she had not changed her eating habits in twenty years. Her increasing weight made her very unfit and she was breathless as she sat down in front of me after climbing the flight of stairs to the surgery. Maggie had come to see me because none of the doctors she had consulted would believe that she was not a 'closet eater'.

Maggie told me that her problem had started just over two years ago when she had been put on hormone tablets to control her menopausal hot flushes. After this her weight began to soar and because she was an android shape she had accumulated fat in the upper part of her body. She had developed a fat face and neck, big arms, a thick trunk and a big protruding abdomen which she tried to conceal under a loose-fitting caftan dress. Her diet had not changed, she had always been a big meat eater and was not partial to sweets or chocolates. Maggie was also battling with high cholesterol and raised blood pressure, which had not been helped by her hormone tablets.

I explained to Maggie that android-shaped women such as herself tended to gain weight easily and that hormone replacement therapy could aggravate this tendency. She had had a hysterectomy and therefore did not require the hormone progesterone, which had been given to her in the form of a large dose of Provera. Synthetic progesterones often have an anabolic action–in other words, they tend to promote an increase in body fat and fluids. Thus, the first step was to stop her progesterone tablets.

Estrogen tablets are more likely to promote weight gain than are the non-oral forms of estrogen such as the estrogen patch, so I switched Maggie to an estrogen patch and stopped her estrogen tablets. To reduce her fatigue I prescribed Magnesium Complete tablets and the Android Body Type (A-Body Type) Figure Control Tablet.

Maggie was started on the Body Shaping Diet for android women (see page 91) and I also asked her to avoid salt and drink ten glasses of water daily. She was greatly relieved that a doctor had finally believed her, and taken her story seriously, as up until then she admitted to me that she seriously thought she was going mad.

Six months later she returned having lost all the excess 44 pounds (20 kg) she had gained after starting hormone replacement therapy. She was back to her 135 pounds (61 kg), had returned to playing tennis, and looked years younger than when I had seen her six months ago.

Maggie had encouraged several of her overweight menopausal girlfriends to follow the Body Shaping Diet for their particular body shape, and all had achieved a successful outcome. She had always been a great cook and popular hostess and was now thinking of setting up a restaurant serving menus from the Body Shaping Diet book in her local town.

CHAPTER FIVE

THE GYNAEOID-SHAPED WOMAN

The gynaeoid shape is the most common female body shape. This type of woman is pear shaped with average to small sized shoulders, variably sized breasts, a small waist and curvaceous buttocks and rounded thighs. She is the voluptuous 'Marilyn Monroe' type and was typically the subject of the great French impressionist painters. She is the model of yesterday and is generally more cuddly and curvy than the lean to skinny stereotyped models of today.

The female hormone estrogen produced by the sex glands or ovaries causes the selective deposition of fat cells in the areas of the breasts, buttocks and thighs. The gynaeoid woman usually has plentiful supplies of estrogen if her ovaries are healthy and indeed if she becomes overweight, she often has excessive amounts of estrogen or a 'hyper-estrogenic state'. Excessive weight will be deposited particularly in the lower half of the body in the feminine areas such as buttocks, pelvis, hips, thighs and eventually the breasts. It is unfortunate that this type of fatty tissue may become uneven and lumpy resulting in tenacious cellulite. We call this type of obesity lower-segment body obesity as it is mainly confined below the waist. The large deposits of fatty tissue are in themselves hormonally active and produce significant amounts of the sex hormone estrogen, in addition to the ovaries pumping out their own monthly surges of estrogen. It is thus easy to understand why an overweight gynaeoid-shaped woman tends to have high levels of estrogen, which will act to further exaggerate the deposition of fat cells in the feminine curvy areas especially the buttocks and thighs. Thus, the gynaeoid woman is often frustrated by her large bottom or 'rear', which may start to droop posterially as she ages. Elizabeth Taylor is a classical gynaeoid woman who has not always managed to keep her estrogenic curves under control.

The dominant hormonal glands in the gynaeoid woman are the ovaries and if you are a gynaeoid woman, as a generalisation, you will normally be fertile and become pregnant easily!

Many gynaeoid women find that when they become significantly over-weight they develop health problems due to excessive estrogen production from their ovaries and fat deposits. There are several organs in the body that are very receptive or sensitive to the effects of the hormone estrogen, especially the breasts and uterus. Estrogen stimulates the breasts and uterus to enlarge and if excessive levels of estrogen are sustained, the breasts may become larger, tender and lumpy and the uterus congested. This latter effect can result in increasingly heavy menstrual bleeding, period pains and increase the risk of fibroids and endometriosis. Gynaeoid women tend to produce more estrogen than progesterone, and this relative excess of estrogen is called "estrogen dominance".

You can now understand how obesity increases the incidence of gynecological problems in women. We also know that obese women have a higher incidence of cancer of the uterus and breasts, partly because of the link between excess weight, hormone imbalance and body organ sensitivity. Gynaeoid women and indeed all women, can reduce their risk of cancer by avoiding obesity—another very good reason to follow the Body Shaping Diet.

CHARLOTTE'S CASE HISTORY

My patient, Charlotte, came to see me in a desperate state. She was obsessed with the appearance of her rather large bottom, which drooped down the back of her thighs. Moreover, Charlotte's bottom was covered with stretch marks, a testimony to the rapid and repetitive weight cycling she had experienced over the last decade. Charlotte was an example of why fast weight loss diets don't work, as they had decreased her muscle mass (lean body tissue) and thus after each crash diet, she found she could tolerate less calories than before. Because she could not stick to such a restrictive diet forever, within a few months of stopping her diet, all her weight loss, plus a few extra pounds would come back. Poor Charlotte had experienced this weight cycling at least a dozen times and was extremely depressed and unmotivated. I told Charlotte that any diet that promises rapid weight loss, would end up making her fatter in the long-term and this was why her bottom and upper thighs had slowly increased over the years.

Charlotte was a typical gynaeoid woman, very much influenced by the monthly fluctuations of her sex hormones, and she found that she gained around 4 pounds before every menstrual period. Premenstrually her food cravings became worse and she binged on creamy foods and sugary quick fixes to cheer and comfort herself. I explained to Charlotte that sugar really becomes a problem when it is consumed in large doses or if it is combined with creamy, fatty foods, such as in the cream buns and layer cakes she wolfed down before her period.

Charlotte had thought that she was jinxed or terribly unlucky as on each of her crash diets she had lost weight first from her face, neck, breasts and abdomen, with her bottom and thighs remaining amazingly the same and full of pouchy cellulite. She was quite angry that no one had ever explained the relationship of body shape to hormonal imbalance and weight excess, as it all seemed so logical to her now. However, I explained it was a new scientific discovery.

Charlotte was eating high-calorie refined creamy foods that were stimulating her dominant ovaries to pump out more estrogen. These foods also caused fat deposition around the lower half of her body and this fatty tissue produced even more estrogen. Her high levels of estrogen caused fat to be laid down around her buttocks and thighs perpetuating her matronly derriere. Poor Charlotte was well down the road to becoming a middle-aged blimp and was frightened she would become like her gynaeoid-shaped mother who had ended up 187 pounds (85 kgs) and 5' 3" (157.5 cm) at the age of fifty-five.

Now that Charlotte understood the link between her gynaeoid shape, hormonal imbalance, and weight problem she was ready to stick to an eating plan that could bring these three factors into harmony. She realised that her binges of creamy and sugary foods were not only making her fat, but also causing fatigue and slowly eroding her health. She was finally craving good health and well-being more than she was craving fat and refined sugar. Charlotte was now ready to begin and stick to the Body Shaping Diet designed for the gynaeoid woman, see page 101.

At this point Charlotte weighed 151 pounds (68 kg) at a height of 5' 2" (157 cm) putting her body mass index at just over 27. I explained to Charlotte that she must avoid the saturated fats found in full-cream dairy products, fried foods, creamy foods, processed foods and takeaway foods. Alcohol was also on the forbidden list as it is very high in calories and contains natural estrogens, which in Charlotte's case were plentiful enough.

Charlotte went off armed with the Body Shaping Diet and an appointment to see me in six weeks. When she returned she bounced into my surgery looking energetic and I noted the big improvement in her complexion. She was delighted with her loss of 7 pounds because for the first time in her life she had lost it from her bottom and thighs. She remarked that, although the rate of weight loss was slower than with her previous crash diets, she was finding it so easy as she was not tired and really enjoyed the nutritious foods in the Body Shaping Diet. Her cravings for junk food had gone and she felt more inclined to exercise regularly. I told her to stick to the diet for the gynaeoid woman and return in eight weeks.

Next time I saw Charlotte she had lost another 9 pounds and was wearing a close-fitting pair of denim jeans and looked slinky and attractive. She was doing it for herself and was more confident. The confidence came from inside Charlotte, as she could see that the cellulite was disappearing from her bottom and thighs and the shape of her body was changing in a way she had always desired.

Twelve months after starting the Body Shaping Diet, Charlotte weighed 118 pounds and could fit into a size ten pair of jeans. She was still a gynaeoid-shaped woman, but her fat cells had re-distributed themselves more evenly throughout her body and were no longer all concentrated in her bottom and thighs. Charlotte liked herself and what's more she liked the feeling of being in control of her body.

CHRISTINE'S CASE HISTORY

Christine, aged thirty-two, had been married for three years and was feeling most dejected by her inability to become pregnant due to the condition of endometriosis. Endometriosis is the gynecological disorder that occurs when the lining of the uterus (endometrium) grows outwards through the fallopian tubes and spills into the pelvic and abdominal cavities where it grows much like a weed. Every month when menstruation occurs, this abnormally sited endometrium bleeds into the pelvic cavity causing painful periods and scarring of the internal organs. Christine had been treated for six months with a powerful drug called Danozol which is masculine in its effect and blocks the action of the female hormone estrogen in the body. Unfortunately, when the Danozol was discontinued, her endometriosis, once again under the influence of estrogen, had started to re-grow causing abdominal and pelvic pains.

Christine was a classical gynaeoid-shaped woman with large curvaceous buttocks and rounded thighs that touched together dimpled with cellulite. She had gained 26 pounds since being married and now weighed 150 pounds (70 kg) at a height of 5' 4" (163 cm), which put her body mass index between 26 and 27. This weight gain was due to her change in lifestyle after being married, when she stopped exercising and began cooking fried and creamy foods to delight her husband. They also drank two or three glasses of wine with each evening meal, adding around 250 calories to the meal.

Christine did not want to re-commence the Danozol as she believed this had contributed to her weight gain and she had come to see me searching for a more natural approach to her obesity and endometriosis. I explained to her that her high-fat, high-calorie diet and excessive weight had caused high levels of estrogen in her body, which had stimulated the growth of the endometriosis. If she were to follow the Body Shaping Diet for the gynaeoid-shaped woman, she would gradually slim down, resulting in lower levels of estrogen and shrinkage of the deposits of endometriosis in her pelvis.

She was most interested to learn that a high-fat diet also caused an increased production of inflammatory chemicals in the body known as prostaglandins. These excessive prostaglandins caused increased inflammation in her uterus and tubes, thus increasing her pelvic pain and congestion.

To reduce inflammation and congestion, I prescribed evening primrose oil 3000 mg daily, calcium 600 mg daily, vitamin A 5000 i.u. daily, vitamin E 1000 i.u. daily and vitamin C with bioflavonoids 2000 mg daily. These nutritional supplements would be slower to act than Danozol, as they did not directly block the production of the body's estrogen, but rather strengthened the immune system, which would gradually control the endometriosis.

I sent Christine off armed with the Body Shaping Diet for the gynaeoid-shaped woman, (see page 101), the prescription for nutritional supplements and the body shaping exercise programme. This exercise programme would not only reduce her large buttocks and thighs, but also improve circulation to the pelvic organs, which is a vital strategy for all women battling with endometriosis.

Christine returned after three months, reporting that her pelvic pain and menstrual periods were much better, however she had lost only 6 pounds in weight, and none from her buttocks and thighs. On further questioning, I discovered that Christine had been doing only two out of the three things I had prescribed. She was taking her nutritional supplements and exercising, but when it came to the Body Shaping Diet, she was following her own variation. Due to pressures from her husband, she was still eating too much fat and creamy foods and found it difficult to cook two meals, one for herself, and one for her husband. I suggested that she cajole her husband into sticking to the Body Shaping Diet with her, with the added reward that by reducing to her normal body weight she would increase her chances of becoming pregnant and having a trouble-free pregnancy. I reinforced that unless she stuck carefully to the Body Shaping Diet for her gynaeoid shape, she would find it very difficult to lose weight from her buttocks and thighs.

Well, this trick really worked and I did not hear from Christine for another year. She popped into the waiting room one day in the full bloom of pregnancy and began enthusiastically telling all the waiting patients that the Body Shaping Diet was a sure-fired way to become pregnant. Not that I designed the Body Shaping Diet to increase fertility, it's primary aim is to re-shape and normalise body weight, but it is fascinating to discover time and time again, that by correcting the diet we not only slim down, but re-balance our hormones and achieve a superior quality of life.

By the way, I forgot to mention that Christine did lose weight from her buttocks and thighs, but became pregnant before the process was complete. The Body Shaping Diet should not be followed during pregnancy, but Christine told me that she would resume it after delivery, as she had never felt better than when she was on it.

REBECCA'S CASE HISTORY

Period pains are a common problem for many women and few realise that they can be related to diet, obesity or lack of fitness. This was so for Rebecca, a classic gynaeoid-shaped woman, who weighed 168 pounds at a height of 5'1", giving her a body mass index of 31. Most of her obesity was in the breasts, buttocks and upper thighs associated with well-advanced cellulite. Rebecca's blood test revealed high levels of estrogen and a tendency towards diabetes (pre-diabetic state). Her uterus was moderately enlarged and congested and tilted backwards (retroverted).

Rebecca was only twenty-three, but she had been overweight for eight years, ever since leaving school and ceasing regular sport. She desperately wanted to lose her large drooping bottom and thick thighs and she was getting nowhere with her severe incapacitating period pains that lasted for two days out of every month. She took large doses of Ponstan or Naprogesic, which dulled the pain, but every month the bleeding seemed to be getting heavier and more painful.

I felt fortunate to be able to assess Rebecca at the young age of twenty-three, as I might otherwise have seen her at age forty, diabetic, very overweight and with an enlarged fibroid uterus or possibly a hysterectomy. As I explained my prognosis to Rebecca, we both realised that she needed to start and stick to a lifetime plan. If Rebecca was going to change her pear shape and eradicate cellulite from her buttocks and thighs, she would need to stick to the Body Shaping Diet for the gynaeoid woman for most of her life. I explained to Rebecca that although the Body Shaping Diet could be used to achieve a so-called classically beautiful figure, this was not the aim for all women and indeed not necessary for happiness or high self-esteem. In her case, I felt it was more important that she lose around 40 pounds to bring her body mass index into the normal range of 19–25, which would give her a weight of around 128 pounds for a height of 5'1". This would reduce her high estrogen levels, greatly reduce her period problems and reverse her pre-diabetic tendency. After these things had been achieved with the Body Shaping Diet, she could then slim down her bottom and thighs further if this was important for her self-esteem.

To prevent period pains, I advised a course of nutritional supplements, namely iron amino acid chelate 100 mg, calcium 800 mg, Magnesium Complete 2 tablets, evening primrose oil 3000 mg (as a daily dose) and the anti-oxidant powder called "Selenomune". I find this a useful programme for many women wanting to reduce period pains and bleeding by natural means. We decided against the oral contraceptive pill as a treatment for period pains, as the synthetic hormones it contained would possibly aggravate her cellulite. For many women, however, the oral contraceptive pill is an excellent way to prevent painful periods. I also started Rebecca on the G-Body Type Figure Control tablets (see page 139). These would help balance her hormones and metabolism, so facilitating weight loss from her buttocks and thighs.

Rebecca went off keen to begin the Body Shaping Diet for her gynaeoid shape and body shaping exercise programme, and promised to return in three months. When she did, her story was most inspiring as she had a significant reduction in her cellulite, had lost 18 pounds, and had been able to cope without the usual mega doses of Ponstan.

One year after our first encounter, Rebecca had achieved her goals and the thing she found surprising was the simplicity and easiness of the Body Shaping Diet. In contrast to other diets she had tried, the Body Shaping Diet did not make her tired, hungry and miserable and she enjoyed inviting friends over to share her meals. She now looked great in a bikini and was free of cellulite at a weight of 124 pounds. From my point of view, I was interested to note that her uterus was no longer enlarged and her blood estrogen and sugar levels were now normal.

CHAPTER SIX

THE LYMPHATIC-SHAPED WOMAN

In the lymphatic-shaped woman, fat is generally distributed evenly all over the body. The head and face are round in shape, the limbs are rather thick and straight up and down. The lymphatic-shaped woman appears more overweight than she really is, due to fluid retention in the fatty layers of the body. This may give a rather pudgy or swollen look to the feet, ankles, hands and wrists.

Fluid retention occurs because the return of blood through the veins in the arms and legs back to the heart is sluggish due to weak valves within the veins and poor muscle tone in the limbs. Fluid also tends to accumulate in the subcutaneous tissues between the skin and the muscle layer because of an inefficient lymphatic system.

The lymphatic system comprises a network of small tubes or vessels that collect subcutaneous fluids and return them to the heart. These lymphatic vessels pass through lymph glands in the groin, abdomen and armpits where the fluid is filtered and cleansed before emptying into the heart. In lymphatic-shaped women, the subcutaneous lymphatic vessels may be deficient in number and quality and may become enlarged and congested. This pre-disposes to puffy, thick limbs which may contain so much excess subcutaneous fluid that on pressing them with the finger tips, a dent is left on the limbs for several minutes. This is called 'pitting edema' by doctors. Lymphatic-type women often use diuretic drugs to try to control this retention of fluid that is such a common problem for them. Diuretic drugs stimulate the kidneys to excrete fluid and salt which gives temporary improvement in fluid retention but does not help the underlying weakness of the veins and lymphatic vessels. Thus, the subcutaneous tissues remain spongy in nature and will swell when fluid once again accumulates in this layer.

The bones are not very obvious in the lymphatic type as they are covered by a thicker layer of fat and fluid. This contrasts with the thyroid type whose bone structure is very evident through their thinner subcutaneous layer. The thyroid woman is the bony type, the lymphatic woman is the cuddly round-type in appearance.

Because the vessel and glands of the lymphatic system tend to be inefficient, problems with the immune system may occur, as the lymphatic system forms an important part of the body's immune system. Thus, problems such as swollen glands, tonsillitis, excessive mucus or allergies may occur, especially if the diet is high in dairy products or processed foods containing artificial chemicals. Excessive mucus and allergies may result in sinusitis, hay fever, sore throats, bronchitis or asthma.

Lymphatic-type women usually crave dairy products which are not metabolised efficiently and result in weight gain and excessive mucus production in the body. To lose excessive fat and fluid, lymphatic types need to follow a diet that is free of dairy products and low in salt (see Body Shaping Diet for lymphatic types, page 105).

A regular exercise programme is vital and the exercises in the body shaping exercise programme are designed to slim down the arms and legs by improving muscle tone and increasing the return of venous blood and lymphatic fluid to the heart. Good muscle tone in the limbs is essential to aid the muscular pump that stimulates the return flow of blood and subcutaneous fluid against the force of gravity upwards to the heart. Swimming, inverted yoga postures, riding an exercise bike, bush walking, power walking and jogging are excellent exercise strategies for lymphatic-shaped women. These types of exercise are often followed by an increased output of urine over the next twenty-four hours, as the kidneys excrete the excessive fluid returned to the heart by the muscles in the limbs during exercise.

Many lymphatic-type women are relatively inactive or sedentary in their lifestyle and have avoided sports during childhood. Indeed they often dislike exercise and competitive sports, as unlike the thyroid types they are not quick movers and they lack the enduring physical stamina of the android types. Their personalities are often relaxed and creative so that they prefer indoor activities such as cooking, painting, reading or entertaining. So it may take some time before a lymphatic-type woman can be coaxed into a regular energetic exercise programme. Unless this is achieved it is very difficult for her to slim down her legs, arms and trunk and replace spongy, subcutaneous tissue with muscle. Lymphatic types will find it difficult to tolerate occupations requiring prolonged standing or sitting in one position all day, as without regular contraction of the limb muscles, fluid will quickly accumulate in the legs and feet.

Lymphatic women have a low metabolic rate and do not burn calories easily, so for them the avoidance of excessive weight is more difficult than for all the other body shapes. If a lymphatic type eats an ice cream it will be converted to fat, whereas the thyroid-type woman will burn up its contained calories far more efficiently. This is somewhat unfair and the lymphatic woman needs to stimulate her metabolic rate with regular exercise and a diet free of dairy products and low in saturated fats, but high in raw fruits and vegetables.

The sluggish metabolism of the lymphatic type can be stimulated by specific foods and nutritional supplements that increase the efficiency of the intracellular biochemistry. This will start to break down excessive fat tissue and improve function of the thyroid gland. To achieve this I recommend that you regularly consume the following foods:

seaweeds	sesame seeds
garlic and onion	green magna
raw vegetable juices	(barley grass extract)
(preferably organically grown)	spices such as chilli
citrus fruits (oranges, lemons,	and fresh ginger, curry,
grapefruits, limes, mandarins)	coriander, tumeric

SPECIFIC NUTRITIONAL SUPPLEMENTS TO BOOST THE METABOLIC RATE OR LIGHT YOUR INTRACELLULAR FIRES ARE:

1. **METABOCEL** is a natural formula designed to stimulate a sluggish metabolism and makes the process of weight loss much easier by speeding it up. The dose of METABOCEL is one tablet, 5 minutes before every meal, with a large glass of water - see page 247

2. **LIVATONE** is a herbal tonic containing liver herbs such as Milk Thistle, dandelion and globe artichoke. The dosage of LIVATONE is 2 capsules twice daily, or one teaspoon of powder twice daily in juices. It is important to improve liver function, as the liver is the main fat burning organ in the body and regulates fat metabolism. Many people cannot lose weight because of sluggish liver function caused by poor diet, drugs and environmental toxins.

3. **L - Body Type Figure Control tablets** are specifically designed to accelerate weight loss in lymphatic body types. They speed up the metabolism, balance the hormones, and cleanse the lymphatic system. The dosage of "L - Body Type Figure Control" tablets is one tablet, three times daily just before meals.

This particular combination of nutritional factors work together, aiding each other in a synergistic way and acting as an intracellular tonic. After taking these nutritional supplements for several months, the lymphatic-shaped woman will find it easier to lose weight while following the Body Shaping Diet and exercise programme. She will have a higher metabolic rate and find that she has more energy to give to the body shaping exercise programme.

The lymphatic-shaped woman will also benefit from foods, herbs and nutritional supplements designed to stimulate her sluggish circulation and lymphatic system. Such supplements will strengthen the weak connective tissues in her blood vessels and swollen lymphatic vessels, reducing vessel fragility. Thus, her capillaries and lymphatic channels will not be so leaky or permeable and fluid will not so readily ooze through vessel walls to accumulate in her spongy subcutaneous layer. As a result, the limbs and abdomen slim down and look less thick and congested. To achieve this effect, I recommend:

1. Raw vegetable juices such as carrot, celery, beet, parsley and ginger.
2. Vitamin C with bioflavonoids—2000 mg daily.
3. Buckwheat in the form of grain, bread and porridge.
4. Magnesium Complete tablets, in a dose of two tablets twice daily, are excellent for reducing fluid retention and muscle cramps in those who use diuretic drugs.

The lymphatic type can also reduce fluid retention by using foods and herbs that are tonics for the kidneys—in other words they stimulate kidney function and the excretion of excess fluid. They can be used as natural diuretics which can help to avoid the excessive use of diuretic drugs. Diuretic drugs can be habit forming and the body becomes more resistant to their effect after prolonged or high dosage.

Natural diuretic foods and herbs are :
1. Celery—fresh stalks and seeds.
2. Parsley—fresh.
3. Dandelion—as coffee, or fresh dandelion leaves in salads.
4. Fruits containing enzymes such as pawpaw and pineapple. The enzymes help to soften the stiff and hardened subcutaneous tissues, thereby enhancing return of retained fluids back to the heart and kidneys. This helps to slim down the limbs.
5. The herbs buchu and horse tail.

The dominant gland in the lymphatic type of woman is the pituitary gland situated at the base of the brain (see page 12). The pituitary gland produces several major hormones and its main role is to control the thyroid gland, the adrenals and the ovaries. The pituitary gland can be considered the master gland of the body—controlling, balancing and orchestrating the overall hormonal state.

Some doctors working in the field of obesity believe that an excess of dairy products in the diet causes an over-stimulated state of the pituitary gland which increases the tendency to obesity, especially in lymphatic types. In some women a high consumption of dairy products stimulates the pituitary gland to overproduce the hormone prolactin. High levels of prolactin disturb the menstrual cycle causing amenorrhea and infertility. The avoidance of dairy products will often cause such high prolactin levels to reduce to normal. The lymphatic diet is free of dairy products. It is true that many lymphatic types of women crave dairy products such as milk, cheese, butter, cream, yoghurt, ice cream and chocolate. These foods are not easily metabolised in lymphatic types and pre-dispose to weight gain and excessive mucus.

Many lymphatic women are Caucasian in ancestry and have fair skin, light-coloured hair and blue or green eyes. If one examines the iris of the eye, it is easy to see the over-burdened lymphatic system in the form of a ring of white dots around the periphery of the coloured iris—this is known as a 'lymphatic rosary' (see diagram 8). After a period of dietary

Diagram 8

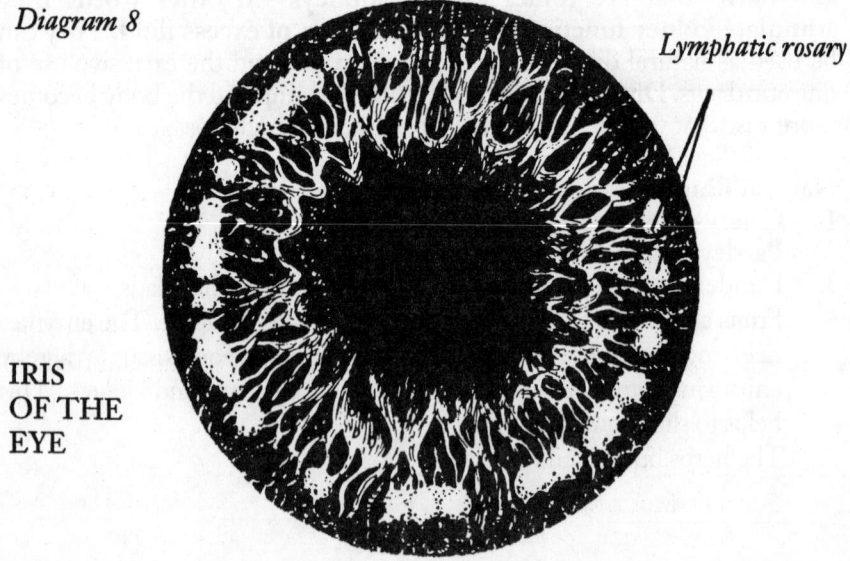

Lymphatic rosary

IRIS
OF THE
EYE

cleansing and elimination of dairy products, this lymphatic rosary will clear and the iris will appear brighter and clearer, reflecting its pure blue or green colour. The cleansing of the eye's irises reflects the internal cleansing going on in the body after a dairy free diet such as the Body Shaping Diet for lymphatic types (see page 105).

PATRICIA'S CASE HISTORY

Patricia had suffered with asthmatic bronchitis for ten years and seemed to be always on antibiotics for another bout of the flu. This made her tired and disinclined to exercise as she felt short of breath and sluggish. She had been slowly gaining weight over the last decade and had put on 15 kg (33 lb) which was distributed evenly over her neck, trunk, buttocks, arms and legs. Patricia weighed 72 kg (159 lb) at a height of 160 cm (5'3"), putting her body mass index at 28.

She was a typical lymphatic shape with thick arms and legs and her wrists and ankle bones were barely visible beneath her subcutaneous tissues swollen with fluid. Patricia complained to me that she felt like a 'blimpy blob' and hated the look and feel of her abdomen and limbs that were spongy and swollen. 'Every spring I swell up, gain weight and feel like I am allergic to the twenty first century,' she said.

True to lymphatic form, Patricia hated strenuous exercise and loved creamy foods high in dairy products. Little did she know that her high ingestion of dairy foods was one of the main reasons that her immune system could not recover sufficiently to overcome her frequent allergies and viral infections. This was evident by the prominent white dots (lymphatic rosary) around the edge of her blue irises and the swollen rubbery lymph glands in her neck.

Patricia was forty years of age and I was pleased to see her at this time knowing that her body was still young enough to respond well to nutritional medicine. If I had seen her ten to fifteen years later, her recovery and weight loss would have been much more difficult and protracted. By this time her immune system may have been damaged so much from her diet, viral infections and repeated courses of antibiotics, that it would be impossible to restore to healthy function. Worse still, she may have ended up with auto-immune diseases or severe asthma requiring large doses of cortisone.

Patricia was motivated to change as she not only looked out of shape, she felt out of shape. I started her on the Body Shaping Diet for lymphatic women and asked her to avoid all dairy products and foods with chemical additives. To reduce fluid retention I asked her to eat fresh celery, parsley, dandelion leaves, pawpaw and pineapple. To improve her resistance to viral infections, I recommended she take Olive Leaf capsules 2 twice daily and Selenomune powder along with one or two fresh garlic cloves everyday. In those unable to tolerate fresh garlic, odourless garlic capsules are a suitable, although slightly less effective alternative.

For the first three months on this programme, Patricia's body and immune system underwent a cleansing and elimination process. Her daily urinary output increased, her bowel actions became looser and more frequent and she had a greater amount of mucus discharge from her sinuses and lungs. There were days when she felt unwell complaining on the other end of the phone of headaches and profound fatigue. I reassured her that this was part of her body's catharsis, and was to be expected while her body was eliminating deeply buried toxic waste products. During these times I encouraged her to stick to the Body Shaping Diet, increase her intake of pure water, and add half a litre of a mixture of raw carrot, beetroot, celery and apple juice made by herself daily with a juice extracting machine.

By the fourth month she had started to notice big changes—she was no longer wheezing, her bronchial mucus had dried up, her limbs were much slimmer and she had lost 9 kg (20 lb) in weight. Now that her energy level was increasing I started her on the body shaping exercise programme and reinforced her need to stick to the Body Shaping Diet and a dairy free diet.

It took twelve months before Patricia fully recovered and regained her lost shape. She was delighted and said that she had been a thin woman trapped inside a fat woman's body for twenty years. She now weighed 57 kg (126 lb) with a body mass index between 22 and 23 and the swollen congested layer of fat that had covered her abdomen and limbs had gone. One could now see her bone and muscle structure and her limbs were no longer thick and shapeless.

JOCELYN'S CASE HISTORY

Jocelyn was an inspiring example of how the Body Shaping Diet and exercise programme can change a woman's life. Two years ago, she had been terribly unhappy battling with a weight problem and severe cyclical fluid retention. She was taking strong diuretic and laxative drugs every day to rid herself of swollen legs and feet. These caused mineral imbalances in her body which resulted in muscle cramps, fatigue and depression.

Jocelyn weighed 78 kg (173 lb) for a height of 155 cm (5'1"), putting her body mass index at 32 and was disgusted with her thick abdomen, arms and legs, so much so that she wore unattractive baggy clothes to hide herself.

She was a typical lymphatic-shaped woman in that she craved dairy products and salty foods. She had been following a high-protein diet in the mistaken belief that if she avoided sugary sweet foods she must lose weight. Jocelyn had cheese on toast for breakfast, a cheese and ham sandwich for lunch and loved spaghetti bolognaise smothered with salty parmesan cheese for dinner. She adored olives, salted peanuts, anchovies and salty fetta cheese. With such a diet she was retaining so much fluid that she was starting to resemble a bloated jelly fish.

I immediately started Jocelyn on the Body Shaping Diet for lymphatic women and asked her to avoid all dairy products and very salty foods. She was instructed to gradually reduce her dose of diuretic drugs by taking them every second day for one month and then every third day thereafter. I advised that she eat foods high in bioflavonoids, vitamin C and rutosides, such as citrus fruits and buckwheat. I prescribed L - Body Type Figure Control tablets and Magnesium Complete tablets to reduce fluid retention and fatigue, and to speed up her weight loss.

For the first two weeks Jocelyn actually retained more fluid, especially in her lower legs and gained 4lb in weight. This was because she had reduced her intake of diuretic drugs resulting in rebound fluid retention. I reassured her that this was only temporary and would pass when her diet and natural diuretics took effect.

Six weeks after she had started the Body Shaping Diet, Jocelyn was starting to feel and look much better. The puffiness had gone from her eyes and feet and she now only needed her diuretic tablets twice a week.

I referred her to a physiotherapist who gave her the technique of lymphatic massage. The physiotherapist massaged her limbs beginning at the fingers and toes and working upwards, so encouraging excess subcutaneous fluid to move up through the lymphatic vessels. This massage also improved circulation to the fatty layer thus stimulating the excretion of waste products from the fat. Jocelyn was also doing the exercises in the body shaping exercise programme to stimulate the muscle pump in her limbs.

A physical metamorphosis started to take place in her limbs and after four months I could see her bony and muscular anatomy defining, where previously there had been layers of swollen fatty tissue. After six months, Jocelyn was a new woman both in appearance and demeanour. She weighed 129 pounds and was wearing body hugging jeans and skirts and was able to wear attractive belts around her now slim and feminine waist. The shy, studious hermit had turned into a social butterfly who was now too busy and full of *joie de vivre* to worry about how she appeared to others.

Two years after our first consultation, Jocelyn met the man of her dreams, at the side of a swimming pool of all places! By this time she looked taut and terrific in a bikini and felt totally relaxed about her uncovered body in public. Thanks to the Body Shaping Diet she had found a way to feel good about herself, improve her health and catch a beautiful man to boot!

CHAPTER SEVEN

THE THYROID-SHAPED WOMAN

The thyroid type has long fine-boned limbs and a slender neck and can be described as lean and rangy. She has the racehorse or greyhound look.

Her dominant gland is the thyroid gland, which is the soft fleshy gland situated in front of the neck or 'adam's apple'. The thyroid gland produces thyroid hormone which stimulates and controls the metabolic rate. The thyroid-shaped woman when in good health has a high metabolic rate and burns up food calories efficiently. Of all the body shapes, the thyroid is the hardest to fatten and generally these types will be able to eat high-calorie and high-fat foods without gaining weight easily.

Thyroid-shaped women are often nervous types and may be described in colloquial terms as 'living on their nerves' or 'highly strung'. They often find it hard to relax and many are workaholics or high achievers. They seem to be always on the go and their high level of mental and physical activity helps to keep them slim.

On the surface, thyroid-shaped women appear to have abundant energy, however it is rather superficial and they lack the enduring stamina of android-shaped women. To keep themselves going, thyroid types often crave quick energy boosters and stimulant substances. Many consume sweets and chocolates, coffee, hot spicy foods, cigarettes, diet pills and other stimulants to boost their energy levels when they start to flag. This makes them feel energetic for several hours until they flag again when more stimulants are required. Such stimulant substances cause their thyroid and adrenal glands to pump out more thyroid hormones and adrenal hormones such as cortisone and adrenalin. These hormones produce a temporary 'high' and raise blood-sugar levels, which enables the thyroid-type woman to continue her frenetic pace.

If these bad habits continue, eventually the thyroid and adrenal glands suffer from a state of depleted exhaustion and weight gain or chronic fatigue occurs. Once the thyroid and adrenal glands become exhausted, the metabolic rate slows down and weight gain occurs. Fat is deposited upon the abdomen and thighs while the lower parts of the limbs remain relatively slim.

Thyroid-shaped women often miss meals preferring to snack on quick fixes such as chocolate, coffee and cakes. They also have the highest incidence of eating disorders such as anorexia and bulimia. Lady Diana, Princess of Wales, was a classical thyroid-shaped woman with long slender limbs. She had the typical thyroid personality and displayed a propensity for eating disorders.

If a thyroid-shaped woman is underweight she will produce lower amounts of estrogen compared to the amounts she produces when her weight falls into the normal range (see table, page 43). She also has relatively less estrogen than the gynaeoid-shaped woman who tends towards estrogen excess. Because the thyroid-shaped woman tends to be low in estrogen or 'hypo-estrogenic', if she becomes underweight she will lose fat first from the estrogen dependent areas of her body, namely her breasts, buttocks and upper thighs. Thyroid-shaped women who fall into the underweight or very underweight range (see graph, page 44), often have such low levels of estrogen, that their menstrual periods become very infrequent or stop completely. This is most undesirable because, if it persists, the chronically low levels of estrogen increase the risk of osteoporosis and cardiovascular disease. This is because our bones, heart and blood vessels require adequate amounts of estrogen to stay healthy.

I always encourage thyroid-shaped women to take care of their thyroid and adrenal glands by avoiding quick-fix stimulants such as sugar, alcohol or cigarettes. These things will make their blood-sugar levels unstable, causing highs and lows in blood sugar—the so-called 'sugar slippery dip' effect. To avoid low blood-sugar levels, they need regular meals containing first-class protein such as fish, meat, dairy products or a combination of grains, nuts, seeds and legumes. The Body Shaping Diet for thyroid women (see page 115) is designed to provide steady amounts of protein and complex carbohydrates to stabilise blood-sugar levels and strengthen the thyroid and adrenal glands. This will avoid the state of chronic thyroid and adrenal exhaustion and resultant obesity that many of these women find themselves in.

Thyroid-shaped women with low levels of estrogen are usually very slim to underweight and may desire to increase the size of their breasts and buttocks—in other words, they may want to look more feminine and curvaceous. To do this, it will be necessary to gain weight and increase the levels of estrogen in the body. The latter can be done with the oral contraceptive pill, which is ideal in younger women requiring regular periods and contraception, or with hormone replacement therapy in older meno-pausal women. If these methods are not suitable another strategy to increase body estrogen levels is to consume foods that have a significant content of natural plant estrogen. Estrogenic substances have been discovered in over three hundred different plants and although they are relatively weak, if they are consumed regularly, they may be helpful in boosting the body's estrogen supply.

FOODS CONTAINING NATURAL ESTROGENS ARE:

linseed	garlic	green beans	red beans
pumpkin	split peas	marrow	cow pea
olives	olive oil	soya bean	bakers' yeast
parsley	chick peas	rhubarb	cherry
corn	oats	barley	rye
wheat	rice	peas	sesame
liquorice	french beans	clover	red clover
apple	fennel	alfalfa	aniseed
hops	sage	corn oil	sunflower
carrots	beetroot	plum	squash
cabbage	soya sprouts	potato	

These foods are high in not only estrogens, but also vitamins, minerals, fatty acids and fibre and are low in saturated fat. Thus there are many good reasons to consume them on a regular basis. There are nutritional formulas available, such as FemmePhase, containing estrogenic herbs and foods as well as vitamins and minerals. For more information call Dr Cabot's Health Line on free call 1888 75 LIVER.

NUTRITIONAL SUPPLEMENTS

There are specific nutritional supplements that act to reduce the tendency to unstable blood-sugar levels and reduce the craving for quick sugar fixes that many women suffer with. Over the years I have encountered thousands of sugarholic and chocaholic women who have been helped with nutritional medicine. Indeed, many of them could not believe how their insatiable cravings for sugar were eliminated, so that they rarely thought of bingeing on sugar, while previously they had been tormented by their need for a quick sugar fix. This sugar addiction is most common in the thyroid-shaped woman, but also occurs to a lesser degree in all the other body shapes.

THE NUTRITIONAL SUPPLEMENTS REQUIRED TO STABILIZE BLOOD SUGAR LEVELS AND REDUCE CRAVINGS FOR SWEETS ARE:

1. "T-Body Type Figure Control" tablets in a dose of one tablet, three times daily before meals.
2. Selenomune powder in a dose of one teaspoon daily in raw vegetable juices
3. Glicemic Balance capsules, in a dose of one capsule, three times daily before every meal.

Thyroid-shaped women suffering with chronic fatigue or obesity will benefit from additional supplements designed to strengthen their thyroid and adrenal glands. These will help the thyroid and adrenal glands to produce steady levels of hormones in the correct balance. The adrenal glands normally produce their peak levels of hormones in the morning, at the start of the day, which is necessary to prepare you for a productive action-packed day. So if you are feeling particularly poor in the mornings, needing strong coffee or a sugar fix, it is a warning that your adrenal glands are not performing well.

SUPPLEMENTS TO HELP THYROID-SHAPED WOMEN WITH CHRONIC EXHAUSTION ARE:

1. Anti-oxidant vitamins e.g. vitamin C 1000 mg daily, beta-carotene 10 mg daily, vitamin A 5000 iu daily, vitamin E 1000 iu daily.
2. Flaxseed Oil capsules in a dose of 2 capsules twice daily with food.
3. Magnesium Complete tablets in a dose of 2 tablets twice daily with food.

These nutritional supplements combined with the Body Shaping Diet and exercise programme will benefit thyroid and adrenal gland function. This will regulate the metabolic rate and start the process of weight normalisation—either weight gain or weight loss, depending on if you are an underweight thyroid shape or an overweight thyroid shape.

These nutritional supplements should be continued in this dosage for three months, thereafter you may take them every second day as a maintenance programme. Once you are feeling entirely well and feel confident with the Body Shaping Diet for thyroid women, you may discontinue the supplements. If, however, you wish to continue them, it is quite safe to do so on a maintenance dose (i.e. every second day).

FUNCTION OF THE THYROID GLAND

When we talk of the function of the thyroid and adrenal glands, we are talking in degrees of relative function. We feel really well and metabolize our food efficiently when our glands are functioning at their optimal level. In some women, the function of the thyroid gland gradually and insidiously becomes sub-optimal. This causes a slowing of the metabolic rate and a reduction in mental and physical activity with resultant weight gain. A blood test done at this time may still show that thyroid gland function falls in the 'normal range' of the general population, although it is often at the lower limits of this normal range. Such women may be told that their thyroid function is 'normal' and to return in twelve months to repeat the test. Most doctors do not accept that treatment is necessary unless the thyroid function falls below the normal range in a blood test. However, what we need to be aware of is that the present state of function of the thyroid gland is often sub-optimal, relative to how it functioned several years ago. Many women, especially thyroid types, are very sensitive to this state of gradual thyroid underactivity and wish to undergo treatment to restore thyroid function before it reaches a level below the normal range in a blood test. In such cases, the nutritional supplements and Body Shaping Diet for the thyroid woman will help to improve thyroid function.

Once blood tests reveal that the thyroid gland is functioning below the normal range, supplementation with thyroid hormone is necessary. A truly underactive thyroid gland will cause the gradual onset of a collection of unpleasant symptoms. Typically these are a general slowing down of all systems resulting in weight gain around the neck and abdomen associated with a general puffiness of the face, hands and legs and dryness of the skin and hair. The body temperature and pulse rate decrease, the voice deepens and constipation occurs. If thyroid hormone replacement is not given a slowness will develop in speech, nervous reflexes and mental activity.

The usual type of thyroid hormone replacement given is Synthroid also known as T4, and this is suitable treatment for the majority of women with an underactive thyroid. After commencing Synthroid, the metabolic rate increases and weight loss and a return of well-being should occur.

THYROID RESISTANCE

A small percentage of women with an underactive thyroid find that replacement with Synthroid does not produce weight loss or a state of well-being. This may be due to a state of thyroid resistance when the body does not respond to Synthroid (T4).

Before T4 can be used by the body, it must be converted in our body cells to another form known as T3, which is the more active and potent form of thyroid hormone. In cases of thyroid resistance the body cannot convert T4 to T3 efficiently. This problem can be overcome by giving thyroid hormone replacement in the form of T3, as well as the conventional T4. T3 can be obtained on prescription under the brand of Tertromel.

If you have an underactive thyroid gland and do not feel well, or are unable to lose weight by taking Synthroid (T4) tablets, you could ask your doctor about the possibility of changing to, or supplementing your Synthroid tablets with Tertromel (T3) tablets. Theoretically, T3 tablets should be more effective in women with a poor response to T4 tablets because they do not need conversion to another form and have a more rapid and powerful effect on the metabolism. Tertromel (T3) tablets are no more expensive than Synthroid (T4) tablets but they need to be given two or three times daily. The starting dose is around 5 micrograms (mcg) twice daily with a gradual increase to around 20–60 mcg daily. Your doctor can adjust the dosage for you to keep you feeling and looking good and to maintain your blood tests for thyroid function within the normal range. It is important that your dosage of thyroid hormone replacement is carefully controlled and you should always be guided by your own doctor in such cases.

MARIA'S CASE HISTORY

Maria came to see me in a most distressed state. She was a beautiful looking girl with black hair and an olive complexion and was a typical thyroid shape with long slim limbs. She had come to see me as a last resort having been to several doctors over the last twelve months seeking help for her underactive thyroid gland.

She had been prescribed thyroid hormone replacement in the form of Synthroid (T4), but it was not helping her symptoms—she remained tired and irritable, her hair and eyebrows were falling out, and she could not lose weight.

On examination, she was definitely carrying some excess weight around her abdomen and thighs and weighed 78 kg (173 lb) at a height of 178 cm (5'10"), giving her a body mass index of approximately 25.

Her doctor had been gradually increasing her dosage of Synthroid (T4) tablets but although her blood tests showed that this dose was resulting in 'normal thyroid function', her symptoms of hair loss and weight gain remained. She was totally frustrated and depressed.

I suggested that she may have a case of thyroid resistance and that we should try reducing her dose of Synthroid (T4) and supplementing it with some Tertromel (T3). Maria was keen to try anything new and so we embarked on the double-pronged strategy of Synthroid (T4) plus Tertromel (T3). I also asked Maria to change her diet and lifestyle and follow the Body Shaping Diet for the thyroid-shaped woman and exercise programme.

Maria returned after three months and was much happier and energetic than she had been during our first encounter. Her hair and eyebrows had stopped falling out and her chronic fatigue was becoming less each day. She was pleased with the Body Shaping Diet as she no longer craved sugar and coffee to keep her going.

After six months on this programme, Maria felt like her old self and was pleased to rediscover her slim thyroid shape at a weight of 145 pounds. It was decided in collaboration with her specialist that she would continue both T4 and T3 in a sufficient dose to keep her blood tests for thyroid function in the normal range.

ZOE'S CASE HISTORY

Zoe's husband brought her to see me as he was increasingly concerned about her low body weight, although Zoe herself was not at all perturbed by her rather anorexic looking body. Zoe was twenty-eight and her weight loss had started after a holiday in Europe, where she had gained 7 kg (16 lb) which prompted her friends to comment on her new shape. Although Zoe had never been obese she was very sensitive to her friend's remarks and she subconsciously decided to lose weight from this point on.

Zoe was a typical thyroid shape with small bones and long skinny limbs and in true thyroid style she relied on stimulants such as cigarettes, chocolates and coffee to keep her going during her busy shifts as a nursing sister in a hospital cardiac unit. She would usually miss breakfast preferring a coffee and cigarette and snacked on a chocolate bar at the mid-morning break. Lunch consisted of a sandwich, however Zoe, being terrified of gaining weight, would ensure that she ate only one quarter of her sandwich and finished off this paltry meal with a coffee and a cigarette.

Zoe's blood sugar levels were understandably quite unstable and around 3 p.m. they would plummet resulting in the need for another chocolate bar. She was a high achiever and very eager to please her colleagues so that she stayed back late at work arriving home around 7.30 p.m. when she would find a tasty healthy meal lovingly prepared by her husband. Despite pleas from her husband, Zoe was lucky to eat half of the food on the plate as during the meal she started to feel guilty and anxious about eating a normal amount of food. The harder her husband tried to encourage her to eat, the more resistant Zoe became, until she finally resorted to hiding some of the evening meal so that her husband would believe she had eaten more than she had.

Zoe's history was typical of an underweight thyroid woman. As her weight loss had continued, her estrogen levels had become lower and lower culminating in the cessation of regular menstrual bleeding. Zoe had not had a period for six months and had lost a lot of weight from the estrogen sensitive areas of her body—namely, her breasts, buttocks and thighs. She definitely looked anorexic with a weight of 47 kg (104 lb) at a height of 170 cm (5'7"), giving her a body mass index of 16.

Due to Zoe's self-imposed calorie restricted diet, which we worked out was around 700 calories per day, her metabolic rate had slowed down as a self-preservation mechanism. This was an automatic reaction of her body to her semi-starvation diet. Due to her slow metabolism her hands and feet felt colder than normal, her pulse rate was slow (under 60) and her skin and hair were dry and unhealthy in appearance.

Despite all this, Zoe felt that everything was fine, as she had now developed in her mind a distorted self-image. Although to all outsiders she looked painfully thin, to herself she was a touch overweight and needed to lose all traces of fat.

I was quite worried about Zoe's future as in the long-term if she continued with her eating patterns, she would have an increased risk of premature osteoporosis and cardiovascular disease secondary to her low body levels of estrogen.

In all anorexic women there is a high resistance to weight gain and normal eating behaviour due to emotional conflicts hidden deep in the subconscious mind. Basically, Zoe suffered from very poor self-esteem and had trouble in asserting her needs. She desperately wanted to enjoy life and to be accepted, but was too frightened to really be herself. Her extremely skinny and unfeminine shape protected her from having to fully involve herself with the outside world and men in particular.

I referred Zoe to a psychologist for in-depth counselling and behaviourial therapy so that we could get her to the point where she wanted to accept a normal eating pattern. In Zoe's recovery plan, the emphasis was on eating for well-being, the restoration of normal estrogen levels and supplements that would maintain normal blood-sugar levels so that she would no longer need to snack on chocolates and candy. The idea of gaining weight and changing body shape was not emphasised strongly, as these things were far too confronting at this point in her recovery. Zoe needed to feel in control of her body and her destiny and I knew that she would remain underweight for some time, at least until she felt ready to change.

My role was to educate her about her body's needs and how her general health and energy could be helped by regular meals containing protein and complex carbohydrates. In the meantime, I could keep a close eye on her weight and metabolism by seeing her every two weeks. In anorexia nervosa there is a significant risk of severe malnutrition and death and I would need to work hard to acquire and keep her trust and confidence.

As I expected, Zoe's weight fluctuated between 103 and 108 pounds for six months. On her fourteenth visit to me, I could see a change in her mental state and demeanour—she was more relaxed and less exacting of herself and was starting to enjoy eating again. On the fifteenth visit she was menstruating and told me that her breasts had been tender that month—a sure sign that her body estrogen levels were returning to normal. She related that her interest in sex had returned and overall she felt more easygoing and less obsessional about controlling everything in her daily life. In other words she was becoming more trusting about the process of life and was taking time to smell the flowers along the way.

After this time, Zoe's weight gain became automatic and she started steadily gaining around half a pound each week. She would occasionally have a bad week and become tense and anxious about work which caused her to miss out on breakfast; during these weeks she would lose around one pound in weight.

Zoe's psychologist taught her meditation and techniques of self-visualisation where she saw herself easily achieving the goals and desires closest to her heart. These things helped Zoe enormously and eighteen months after our first encounter she had reached a weight of 55 kg (121 lb), putting her body mass index at 19. This was just slightly under the desirable weight range for her height and small skeletal frame. I was quite happy with this as Zoe's estrogen levels, menstrual cycle and general metabolism were all back to normal. Zoe was once again enjoying life and now that she had more energy she started the body shaping exercise programme to tone up her arms and legs.

Zoe's case history is typical of many women with anorexia nervosa that I have seen over my years in clinical practice. Anorexia nervosa is a form of self-imposed semi-starvation and is more common in thyroid-shaped women. It needs to be handled with great sensitivity, compassion and skill if a cure is to be long lasting.

CLANDESTINE'S CASE HISTORY

Clandestine was a model for a fashion house and was paid handsomely to model a range of swimwear. She had a thyroid-shaped figure with a long fine neck, smallish bone structure and the longest pair of legs I had ever seen.

In typical thyroid style, Clandestine was addicted to stimulants—she craved caffeine, cigarettes, chocolates and hot spicy Asian foods. She was also addicted to diet pills which gave her a temporary stimulus and helped her to avoid bingeing on chocolate.

Not surprisingly, Clandestine suffered extreme mood changes and energy highs and lows, which made it difficult for her to exercise and keep her muscles toned sufficiently to flatter her swimwear range. She was worried by the slow accumulation of fat around her abdomen and upper thighs and came to me seeking help to regain her trim muscular form.

To keep her mood changes under control, Clandestine's doctor had prescribed anti-depressant drugs, however their sedative effects were not tolerated by Clandestine's thyroid-type personality, which was accustomed to feeling stimulated and not sedated. These anti-depressant drugs also caused her appetite to increase so she had been quick to discard them.

I explained that if we kept her levels of blood sugar, thyroid and adrenal hormones steady, instead of their present wild fluctuations, we could stop her mood swings and fatigue. This would then enable Clandestine to easily resist her cravings for sugar, coffee and stimulant diet pills.

To achieve these goals Clandestine was started on the Body Shaping Diet for thyroid-shaped women and the body shaping exercise programme. This particular diet contains complex carbohydrates and first-class protein in each meal (see menus page 112) which stabilise blood sugar levels. The Body Shaping Diet for thyroid women is high in protein, minerals such as calcium, magnesium and iodine and also contains an abundance of estrogenic foods. These ingredients are beneficial for the function of the thyroid gland and help to maintain strong youthful bones.

Clandestine was asked to avoid her binges on sugar, coffee, chocolate, cigarettes and very hot spicy meals, as in the long-term these stimulants would exhaust her thyroid and adrenal glands making it very difficult for her to lose weight. To aid her resolution, I prescribed the T-Body Type Figure Control tablets, one three times daily and Glicemic Balance capsules, one three times daily. These would stabilise her blood-sugar levels and greatly reduce her cravings for stimulant foods and drugs.

To reduce her unpleasant mood changes which alternated from depression and fits of crying to extreme anger and aggression, I prescribed some single amino acids to be taken with a glass of orange juice at night. These consisted of tryptophan 800 mg, and glutamine 400 mg. To these I added Magnesium Complete tablets, in a dose of two tablets with the evening meal. These nutritional supplements would re-balance the chemicals in her brain cells (neuro chemicals) and promote a more stable and efficient mode of mental functioning.

As thyroid types tend to be driven and burn the candle at both ends, I emphasised the need for eight hours sleep at night, time for relaxation and time to follow the Body Shaping Diet plan.

Because Clandestine was only 12 pounds overweight, that is as far as keeping her modelling job was concerned, it only took her five weeks on the Body Shaping Diet to lose the excess pounds from her abdomen and thighs. She was very grateful for the nutritional supplements because they had stopped her horrible moods and angry outbursts which were ruining her relationships. They had also enabled her to give up diet pills, coca cola and chocolate, and she thought it fabulous that one could follow a tasty diet, not feel tired and deprived and still lose weight! I replied, 'Simply elementary, my dear. Re-balance the hormones and body biochemistry and the weight takes care of itself!'

MIGRAINES

One other point I would like to mention is that migraine headaches occur more frequently in thyroid-shaped women, especially those with the typical thyroid high-achieving or driven personalities. In thyroid-type women who suffer migraines, it is prudent to avoid foods containing the amine called 'tyramine'. Such foods are wine (especially red), beer, chocolate, lima and Italian beans, mature or hard yellow cheeses and indeed all cheeses (except for cottage cheese), chicken liver, raisins, plums, beef liver, chicken skin, herring, fish marinades, dried mackerel, dried sardines, sausage, marmite, bonox, soy sauce, meat extracts, very ripe bananas, pineapple, eggplant, tomato, walnuts, pecan nuts. This is because tyramine can cause the blood vessels in the brain to constrict and then swell resulting in migraine headaches.

STRATEGY OF THE BODY SHAPING DIET

STEP ONE—WEIGHT LOSS
STEP TWO—MAINTENANCE
RECIPES

Strategy of the Body Shaping Diet

The Body Shaping Diet is simple and easy to follow and uses a two-step strategy.

STEP ONE

WEIGHT LOSS

STEP ONE of the diet allows you to have 1000 calories (4200 kJ) each day to achieve maximum weight loss. You will enjoy nutritious and economical meals that require minimal preparation.

Stay within the guidelines for your body type, selecting only those foods recommended and avoiding completely the 'undesirable foods'.

In **STEP ONE** is a range of sample menus for breakfast, lunch and dinner, suited to each body type, from which you may select meals freely. They are calculated at 1000 calories per day.

Because the basic strategy includes a high intake of carbohydrate foods such as wholegrains and starchy vegetables you will find the meals very satisfying. You will not experience fluctuations in blood-sugar levels which can leave you tired, moody and excessively hungry.

Each body type will have its individual danger periods when you will be tempted to snack. This is explained in detail in later chapters. Have some raw celery, carrot or apple on hand for these occasions.

No other foods should be eaten at these times or weight loss will be slowed down.

While on **STEP ONE** of the programme it is most beneficial for you to follow the exercise programme. This will speed weight loss by burning fat and toning muscle tissue. Positive results will show very quickly and you will look and feel lighter with an increase in energy and vitality.

You may wish to keep a food diary, where you write down all foods eaten each day.

> **Weigh and measure yourself once a week at the same time of day and keep a record. Take measurements of your bust, waist, hips, buttocks, thighs and upper arms. Some weeks, as your body shape and metabolism are changing, you may not lose pounds but you will lose inches.**

When you have reached your desired body weight move straight on to **STEP TWO**—the Maintenance Programme designed specifically for your body shape

STEP TWO

WEIGHT MAINTENANCE

Our maintenance strategy allows you to increase your caloric intake to suit your individual requirements. We have included a range of sample menus for breakfast, lunch and dinner calculated at approximately 1400 calories (5880 kJ) per day.

Some women will find this is too high and may need to keep their caloric intake at 1200 calories (5040 kJ) per day to maintain a desirable weight. Others who exercise consistently may need a little more than 1400 calories (5880 kJ) each day.

While following our maintenance strategy you will enjoy the freedom of introducing some healthy desserts (see recipe section) into your diet. You will also increase your fruit and carbohydrate intake.

Staying within the guidelines for your body shape (beginning on page 92) makes it easy for you to maintain your desirable weight and to continue to look and feel healthy and vital.

GENERAL GUIDELINES FOR ALL BODY SHAPES

* **Drink 8 glasses of water daily.** This includes soda water, mineral water and herbal teas.

* **Chew your food well.** This is important for the digestion of all foods, particularly fruit, raw vegetables and grains. The nutrients in these foods are surrounded by undigestible cellulose membranes which need to be broken in order for you to utilise the nutrients locked inside. Chewing also triggers the secretion of enzymes which are necessary for the breakdown and utilisation of your food. Food that has been chewed well will not irritate the lining of the stomach or the intestines and is digested with ease.

* **Do not drink with meals.** It is important not to interfere with digestion by washing down undigested food with drinks. Try to have your fluids about half an hour before or after meals.

* **Eat in a relaxed environment.** If you are stressed while eating **you** are more likely to rush your food which will lead to difficult digestion and possibly discomfort.

• **Try to eat early in the evening.** Going to bed with a full stomach is often a major contributor to poor sleep patterns. There may also be a large time gap between lunch and dinner and this can lead to binge eating if your blood sugar level is allowed to drop too low.

• **Never skip breakfast.** There are no excuses for avoiding breakfast as it recquires minimal preparation. You must provide nutrients, fibre and energy to your body in the mornings in order to remain physically and mentally alert, and to avoid mood swings.

• **Shop wisely.** Make sure your refrigerator and pantry is well stocked with healthy food choices. The most economical way to shop is to buy fresh food . The packaged and processed foods are the ones that are often unhealthy, unnecessary and expensive.

• **Maintain a positive attitude.** Set yourself realistic goals that you are able to achieve and try not to dwell on past failures. Live in the present moment.

• **Stay close to nature.** Select foods which do not contain chemical additives, colours or preservatives.

BREAKFAST

The first meal of the day is designed to increase your metabolic rate and to **BREAK** the twelve-hour **FAST** that has occurred overnight.

You should be rested and ready to eat a light but substantial meal that contains all the nutrients and energy to sustain the morning's activities.

Remember, while on **STEP ONE** of the Body Shaping Diet, even at breakfast you must take care to eat the correct balance of foods for your body shape.

If you prefer to design your own menu, simply check the amount of calories recommended for your body type, follow your guidelines and create a breakfast that includes a carbohydrate food like cereal or toast, some protein such as low-fat dairy products, eggs, fish, soy milk etc, a serve of fruit (see list page 204) and a beverage of your choice.

Eating breakfast will reduce the temptation to snack mid-morning.

LUNCH

Lunch can vary greatly according to your daily routine. Whether it simply consists of a salad sandwich or a more elaborate business lunch, **by making the right choices it will always be possible to follow your guidelines and achieve weight loss.**

Try not to eat a late lunch or you will experience a drop in blood sugar. If this happens it can turn someone with tremendous willpower into a creature who will devour anything to obtain a quick sugar fix.

If designing your own lunch menu, check your caloric allowance for lunch and the guidelines for your body shape.

Have a small serve of protein (page 199) and adequate carbohydrate (page 192). Always include lots of green leafy vegetables or salad to assist with digestion and to add nutrients. You may eat your fruit serve with lunch or save it for an afternoon snack.

MAIN MEAL OF THE DAY

Whether you have your main meal at lunch or in the evening it must include a serve of a complete protein food, carbohydrate food and green vegetable or salad.

PROTEIN

Meat 3.5 ounces. Must be lean and fresh with all visible fat removed before cooking. Approximately **180 cal/**750 kJ. DO NOT FRY.

Chicken 3.5 ounces. Remove all visible fat and skin before cooking. DO NOT FRY. Serving size is approximately ½ chicken breast which is about **125 cal/**525 kJ.

Fish 3.5 ounces. Approximately **100 cal/**420 kJ. DO NOT FRY.

Soy beans (cooked). 1 cup is approximately **200 cal/**840 kJ.

The only legumes which are complete protein foods are soy beans. Incomplete proteins are chick peas, navy beans, borlotti beans, red kidney beans, lentils, brown rice, millet and barley. These should be combined to form a complete protein meal, such as mixing chickpeas and tahini (sesame paste) to make hoummos which is a complete protein. Or make a complete protein meal with Dahl (recipe page 171) and rice and vegetables.

Your recommended serving size for cooked legumes is 1 cup.

At your main meal, as well as your protein, have **two or three serves of starchy vegetables.** Choices are as follows:

1 SERVE

= 1 small jacket potato   **(90 cal/378 kJ)**
= 2 scoops* sweet potato   **(65 cal/273 kJ)**
= 1 scoop* pumpkin   **(25 cal/105 kJ)**
= 1 medium beetroot   **(22 cal/92 kJ)**
= ½ cup carrots   **(17 cal/71 kJ)**
= ½ cup cauliflower   **(20 cal/84 kJ)**
= ¼ cup peas   **(20 cal/84 kJ)**
= 1 medium corn cob   **(62 cal/260 kJ)**
= ½ large parsnip   **(50 cal/210 kJ)**

* When I use the term 'scoop' I am referring to icecream scoop size.
If you are having pasta or rice with your meal, it replaces your serves of starchy vegetable. This means that you are allowed to eat the pasta or rice with some protein and unlimited green vegetable or salad.

CARBOHYDRATE

OR

1 SERVE = 2–3 STARCHY VEGETABLES

OR

= 1 CUP COOKED PASTA (approx. 200 cal/840 kJ)

OR

= ¾ CUP COOKED RICE (approx. 180 cal/756 kJ)

ALWAYS SERVE WITH UNLIMITED GREEN VEGETABLE OR SALAD. These greens provide necessary nutrients and fibre and need to be eaten every day. Always have at least two serves of green vegetable. They are very low in calories and will speed your weight loss.

Try not to have bread with the main meal of the day.

Your fruit serve may be eaten at any time.

THE WEIGHT PLATEAU

While following the Body Shaping Diet, there will be times when your weight will stabilize. According to the scales it may not change for a number of weeks.

Maintain your enthusiasm and know that this is a period of transition.

Keep in mind that your body is undergoing a process of change. It takes time to break down stubborn areas where fat cells have been deposited. At the same time your increased exercise helps to build muscle tissue which is heavier than fat.

While your body changes shape, weight loss may stand still periodically. While in a plateau, you may not lose any weight for six to eight weeks. This does not mean that the diet is NOT working, because during these times your metabolism and the structure and function of your fat cells is changing.

If you can stick with your program during these frustrating plateaus, weight loss will surely resume, often at a faster rate than before. People who cannot cope with the plateau phase of weight loss are usually weighing themselves too often and are too obsessed or "hung up" with their weight. Simply concentrate on your eating program and becoming healthy, and look to the end of the road – do not fall into a pothole. Many people who lose patience during the plateau phase, become "yo yo dieters" and follow many types of diets, but in the end they become very overweight and dissatisfied. Patience is a virtue here, and it can be a good idea to throw those bathroom scales away during these times.

ANDROID SHAPE EATING PLAN

If you fall into this category you will find that many weight-loss diets don't work for you, especially if they encourage a high intake of saturated and a reduction of bread, cereals and starchy vegetables.

Your diet needs to be high in raw fruits, fresh vegetables and wholegrains. Protein should come from pulses, legumes, nuts, seeds, fish and low-fat dairy products. You may also include some free range chickens and eggs in your weekly regime and occasionally lean red meats.

PLANNING YOUR EATING PROGRAMME

You will start the day with a light, nutritious breakfast containing fruit, cereal or wholegrain toast and low-fat dairy products or low-fat soy milk.

> A semi-vegetarian diet sits well with you and I have included some vegetarian meals in your sample menus. You will find the vegetarian recipes are very easy to prepare and will supply you with adequate first-class protein.

If you become very overweight, you may face some serious health risks such as diabetes, cardiovascular disease, high blood pressure and high blood cholesterol. These have been considered by me while planning your eating programme.

Lunch is also kept light with an emphasis on soups, salads, bread, grains, seeds, nuts, pasta, pulses, beans and fruit. This will keep your appetite under control and re-balance the glands in your body. You cannot alter your adrenal dominance by simply reducing animal products and salt. You must also eat foods to stimulate the liver and so improve your ability to metabolize cholesterol and breakdown excessive steroid hormones.

Cereals, grains and low-fat dairy products stimulate the thyroid and pituitary glands. This will improve your metabolic rate, regulate hormonal imbalance and open up your creative thought processes.

Late afternoon is often the time when you experience fatigue and hunger. Cheese, crackers and salted peanuts are not the answer, even though the craving for these foods will be strong. You must also avoid the temptation to have an alcoholic drink. This will add unnecessary and useless calories and place added stress on your liver.

As a late afternoon snack have some raw vegetables, such as celery and carrots with an avocado dip, or a small bowl of vegetable soup, or a handful of raw almonds. You will not have to wait long for your dinner which will be substantial and very satisfying.

ANDROID GUIDELINES

FOOD GROUPS	DESIRABLE FOODS	UNDESIRABLE FOODS
Grains, cereal, bread and pasta	Wholegrains such as brown rice, millet, barley, wheat, rye, rolled oats, corn, buckwheat. Bread crispbread, flour and pasta containing these wholegrains	Highly refined and bleached white flour products such as white bread, packaged cakes and biscuits. Avoid products made from bakers' flour or breadmaking flour.
Pulses and beans	All beans, lentils and peas. Tofu and houmos. All bean sprouts.	
Meat, chicken, game and fish	Fresh and tinned fish. Free range chickens, turkeys and eggs. Occasional lean red meats.	Shellfish and oysters. Battery hens and eggs. Offal meat. Anchovies, processed meat, bacon, sausages, fried meats. Roast meat dinners.
Dairy products	Low-fat yoghurt. Sheep and goats' yoghurt. Rice milk	All full-cream dairy products, including chocolate, cream, cheese, butter and icecream. Coconut milk.
Fruit and vegetables	All fresh or dried fruits, tinned fruit in natural juice. A wide variety of fresh vegetables.	Fruit in sugar syrup, Glacé fruit.

ANDROID GUIDELINES

FOOD GROUPS	DESIRABLE FOODS	UNDESIRABLE FOODS
Nuts and seeds	Unsalted raw nuts and seeds. Tahini and raw nut pastes.	Peanuts and salted nuts. Coconut. Peanut butter.
Fats and oils	Small amounts of olive, linseed and canola oil.	Copha, dripping, ghee butter, suet and lard, margarine.
Beverages	Water: 6–12 glasses. Mineral and soda water. Cereal beverages. Some herb teas. Tea (tannin-free best) 1–2 cups coffee/day.	Carbonated soft drinks. Mix-up cordials. Malted milk drinks. Alcohol. Tannin-rich tea. Chocolate drinks.
Miscellaneous	Very small amounts of honey, sugar or molasses.	Refined sugars and products containing sugars. MSG–621. Salt and salty foods. Artificial additives, preservatives and colours.

STEP ONE

WEIGHT LOSS FOR THE ANDROID BODY SHAPE

On waking have a large glass of water with a squeeze of lemon or lime juice.

BREAKFAST

Select any **one** of the following choices.

EACH SELECTION = APPROXIMATELY 250 CAL/1050 kJ

* ¾ cup fresh berries, 7 ounces low-fat natural yoghurt, 1 dessertspoon LSA (see page 209). Cup of herbal tea.

* one ounce cereal (see page 195), 3½ ounces low-fat calcium-enriched milk, ½ tablespoon each lecithin and LSA (see page 209), 6 medium strawberries.

* 2 slices dry wholemeal toast with ¼ cup cottage cheese, sliced tomato and alfalfa sprouts. 1 nectarine.

* ¾ cup cooked rolled oats with 3½ ounces low-fat calcium-enriched milk, soy milk or Rice milk and ½ cup of sliced strawberries and banana, 1 heaped teaspoon each of LSA (see page 209) and wheatgerm.

* 1 Wholemeal Pancake (recipe page 182) with lightly cooked mushrooms, tomato, bean sprouts and fresh dill, gently mixed into ¼ cup ricotta cheese. 1 wedge rockmelon.

* 1 slice dry wholemeal toast with ½ cup salt-reduced baked beans, fresh tomato slices, alfalfa sprouts and fresh parsley. 1 kiwifruit.

* Your choice of a serve of fresh fruit blended with 7 ounces low-fat calcium-enriched milk or Rice milk, ice cubes and 1 heaped teaspoonful of lecithin and wheatgerm. 1 slice raisin or fruit loaf.

* 1 poached or boiled egg with 1 slice dry wholemeal toast, served with sliced tomato, sprouts and ground black pepper. 7 ounces fresh orange juice.

* 1 Apple and Oatbran Muffin (recipe page 182), 1 serve fresh fruit of your choice. Cup of herbal tea.

* 2 slices dry wholemeal toast topped with one ounce chopped sardines in spring water (drained) and freshly chopped chives and parsley. 1 serve fresh pawpaw.

* 1 toasted wholemeal muffin spread with a little cottage cheese and topped with lightly cooked fresh mushrooms and crushed garlic. Sprinkle with roasted sesame seeds. 1 sliced kiwifruit and 6 strawberries.

* 1 slice dry wholemeal toast topped with ¼ avocado, fresh tomato slices, chopped chives and freshly ground black pepper. 2 wedges rockmelon or honeydew.

LUNCH

Select any **one** of the following choices

EACH SELECTION = APPROXIMATELY 350 CAL/1470 kJ

* Guacamole (recipe page 153), served with sticks of mixed fresh raw vegetables such as radish, fennel, carrot, zucchini, capsicum, celery and broccoli florets. 1 serve fresh fruit.

* ½ pocket bread with 1 Falafel (recipe page 170), 1 tablespoon Hummus (recipe page 154), lettuce and Tabbouli Salad (recipe page 155). 1 banana.

* Wholemeal bread roll with fresh green salad, tomato, raw grated beetroot and ¼ medium avocado. ½ custard apple.

* Italian Noodle Soup (recipe page 146), green salad with No Oil Dressing (recipe page 148), 2 wholemeal Premium crackers. 1 serve fresh fruit or juice.

* 3½ ounces red salmon and ¼ cup cottage cheese with a large garden salad and 1 medium cooked beetroot. 2 rockmelon wedges.

* 2 sesame Ryvita with ⅓ cup ricotta cheese, 2 ounces drained, chopped sardines, fresh tomato slices, onion and fresh parsley. 2 slices fresh pineapple.

* Pasta Salad (recipe page 157), 1 jacket potato. 7 ounces apple juice.

* Minestrone Soup (recipe page 145), garden salad with beetroot, 1 wholemeal bread roll. Small bunch of grapes.

* Quick Curried Eggs (recipe page 172), garden salad. 1 serve fresh fruit or juice.

* Asparagus Vinaigrette (recipe page 155), 1 jacket potato with Mock Sour Cream (recipe page 148), 2 wholemeal Premium crackers. 4 lychees or rambutans.

* Low-Calorie Cannelloni (recipe page 174), garden salad, 1 medium-sized cooked beetroot. 1 serve fresh fruit or juice.

* Bowl of Pumpkin Soup (recipe page 146), 2 slices rye bread, Mushroom and Snow Pea Salad (recipe page 159). 1 cup watermelon balls.

EVENING

Select any **one** of the following choices.

EACH SELECTION = APPROXIMATELY 400 CAL/1680 kJ

* 3½ ounces grilled white fish with Tomato Salsa (recipe page 151), 1 jacket potato with 1 dessertspoon of Mock Sour Cream (recipe page 148) green salad with No Oil Dressing (recipe page 148). ½ cup fruit salad.

* Papaya and Chicken Salad (recipe page 161), ½ cup cooked brown rice, Cucumber Salad (recipe page 161).

* Green Vegetable Plate with Dukkah (recipe page 156), 1 cup Dahl (recipe page 171), ½ cup cooked brown rice. ½ sliced banana with 1 passionfruit.

* 2 small taco shells filled with Quick Mexican Beans (recipe page 171), fresh chopped tomato, shredded lettuce, alfalfa sprouts, low-fat natural yoghurt and Chilli Sauce (recipe page 149). 1 serve fresh fruit of your choice.

* Open Soy or Lentil Burger (recipe page 170) on a wholemeal bread roll with salad and sprouts, Chilli Sauce (recipe page 149). 2 slices fresh pineapple.

* Braised Steak (recipe page 165), ½ cup cooked brown rice. Fresh fruit of your choice.

* Alternative Cannelloni (recipe page 174), 1 scoop sweet potato, ½ cup carrots, ½ cup cauliflower, ¼ cup green peas, ½ cup lightly cooked mushrooms. 1 serve fresh fruit.

* Baked Fish with Fruit Filling (recipe page 163) dry baked potato with Mock Sour Cream (recipe page 148), garden salad.

* 1 cup cooked spaghetti with Quick Pesto Sauce (recipe page 150), garden salad with No Oil Dressing (recipe page 148). 1 serve fresh fruit.

* Chicken and Mushroom Pie (recipe page 167), 2 scoops potato mashed with finely chopped onion and parsley, ½ cup carrots, ½ cup cabbage, 2 brussels sprouts. 1 serve fresh fruit.

* 3 ½ ounces grilled veal with Napolitana Sauce (recipe page 175), 1 small jacket potato and garden salad. 1 serve fresh fruit.

* Cabbage Rolls (recipe page 168), 2 scoops sweet potato, ½ cup carrots, ¼ cup of peas and ¼ cup of green beans. 1 serve fresh fruit.

GYNAEOID SHAPE EATING PLAN

From clinical experience I have observed that gynaeoid-shaped women usually skip breakfast or simply enjoy a 'tea and toast'-type breakfast. They will often comment that once they start to eat a heavy meal in the mornings, they find it hard to stop and will 'binge' all day. Whereas if they eat lightly in the morning and have a small lunch they usually feel much lighter and are able to keep their weight under control.

They seem to save up all day and let loose in the evening when some women eat in excess of 1000 calories (4200kJ) just having dinner - with wine, followed by dessert, then a hot drink with a couple of biscuits, then supper, then for some, the evenings are a total disaster.

Is it any wonder that they often sleep badly and wake up tired? They feel bloated and heavy and are usually prone to constipation due to an overindulgence of food in the evenings and no fiber for breakfast to help push through last night's meal.

I encourage you to keep breakfast and lunch light, as long as they are nutritious and provide your body with the necessary fiber. You will see from the sample menus provided that this is encouraged.

You must never skip breakfast because your first danger period for snacking is late morning. Without breakfast your blood-sugar levels will be low and you will be 'hanging out' for a quick fix at morning teatime. This is when you are more likely to go for biscuits or cake with coffee or tea. Instead, you should be having a glass of water, natural mineral water or herb tea with a serve of fruit if you are hungry.

Our lunchtime menus are satisfying and nutritious. They are flexible and easy, whether at home or at work ,or if you have to buy lunch.

Try to have dinner early in the evening so the gap from lunch to dinner is not too long.

If you must eat late, save a fruit serving for early evening or chew some raw salad vegetables until dinner is ready. They are low in calories and easily digested.

Your evening meal is the largest of the day because this is when your metabolism is most active. You enjoy eating in the evenings and so I have designed an eating plan that presents you with a generous and tasty meal that will not leave you hungry.

Your second danger period is late at night when you tend to look for comfort foods, however our evening meals are especially designed to satisfy you so that your cravings at this time are minimal. If you must eat something simply stick to raw fruits and vegetables.

GYNAEOID GUIDELINES

FOOD GROUPS	DESIRABLE FOODS	UNDESIRABLE FOODS
Grains, cereals, bread and pasta	Wholegrains, such as brown rice, corn, rye wheat, buckwheat, oats millet and barley. Bread, pasta containing these wholegrains.	Highly refined and bleached white flour products such as white bread, packaged cakes and crispbread, flour and biscuits. Avoid products made from bakers' flour or breadmaking flour.
Pulses and beans	Most beans, lentils and peas. (Soak dried beans overnight in water). Tofu and houmos.	Soy beans and bean sprouts are high in plant estrogens, so eat in moderation.
Meat, chicken, game and fish	Choose lean cuts of red meats and trim off fat before cooking. Free range chickens, turkeys and eggs. Fresh and tinned fish.	Processed meats, bacon, sausages, fried foods. Roast meat dinners. Skin on poultry. Battery hens and eggs. Offal meats. Anchovies.

GYNAEOID GUIDELINES

FOOD GROUPS	DESIREABLE FOODS	UNDESIREABLE FOODS
Dairy products	Low-fat milk and yoghurt. Sheep and goats' yoghurt. Rice milk.	Full-cream dairy products including butter, cream, ice-cream, cheese.
Fruit and vegetables	All fresh and dried fruits, tinned fruit in natural juice. A wide variety of fresh vegetables.	Fruit in sugar syrup, glace fruit.
Nuts and seeds	Unsalted raw nuts and seeds. Tahini and raw nut pastes.	Peanuts and salted nuts. Peanut butter.
Fats and oils	Small amounts of olive, linseed and canola oil. Tahini, nut spreads avocado	Copha, dripping, ghee butter, suet and lard. Peanut, sunflower, corn, safflower and corn oils.
Beverages	Water: 6-12 glasses. Mineral and soda water. Cereal beverages. Herb teas. Tannin-free tea. 1-2 cups coffee/day	Carbonated soft Drinks. Mix-up cordials. Malted milk drinks. Alcohol Tannin-rich tea. Chocolate drinks.
Miscellaneous	Very small amounts of Honey, sugar or molasses.	Refined sugars and products containing sugar. MSG-621 Salt and salty foods. Artificial additives, Preservatives and colors.

WEIGHT LOSS FOR THE GYNAEOID BODY SHAPE

On waking have a large glass of water with a squeeze of lemon or lime juice.

BREAKFAST
Select any one of the following choices.
EACH SELECTION = APPROXIMATELY 250 CAL/1050 kJ

* 2/3 cup cooked brown rice, 3½ ounces low-fat calcium-enriched milk or soy milk, 1 dessertspoon wheatgerm. 6 small or 3 large strawberries.

* ¾ cup cooked rolled oats, 3½ ounces low-fat calcium-enriched milk, skim milk,or low-fat soy milk, sprinkle with roasted sesame and sunflower seeds. ½ large or 1 small banana.

* 1 poached or boiled egg, 1 slice dry wholegrain toast, topped with fresh chopped parsley, 2 slices fresh tomato, snow pea sprouts. 7 ounces fresh orange juice.

* Fruitshake - your choice of a serve of fresh fruit, blended with 7 ounces skim milk, low-fat calcium-enriched milk, low-fat soy milk or Rice milk, ice cubes and 1 heaped teaspoon each of LSA (see page 209) and wheatgerm. 1 slice of raisin or fruit loaf.

* 2 slices dry wholegrain toast topped with 1/4 avocado, sprinkled with lemon juice and ground black pepper.

* 1 ounces breakfast cereal (list page 195), 3½ ounces skim milk, low-fat calcium-enriched milk or low-fat soy milk or Rice milk, 1 dessertspoon wheat-germ. 1 serve fresh fruit.

* 2 Wholemeal Pancakes (recipe page 182), ½ sliced banana, 1 passionfruit and 1/4 pawpaw.

* 2 slices dry wholemeal toast spread with 1 tablespoon Hummus (recipe page 154), add sliced tomato topped with finely chopped parsley. 7 ounces freshly squeezed orange juice.

* 1 Banana and Pecan Muffin (recipe page 183). 1 serve fresh fruit of your choice. Cup of herbal tea.

* 1 dry toasted wholemeal muffin topped with fresh tomato, parsley and freshly ground black pepper. 1 serve fresh pawpaw.

* 1 slice dry wholemeal toast with ½ cup salt-reduced baked beans, fresh tomato slices and shredded lettuce. 1 wedge rockmelon.

* Lightly cook ½ cup of fresh mushrooms with a little crushed garlic and serve on 2 slices wholemeal toast, thinly spread with ricotta cheese, sprinkle with roasted sesame seeds. 1 serve fresh fruit or juice.

LUNCH

Select any one of the following choices.

EACH SELECTION = APPROXIMATELY 300 CAL/1260kJ

* 2 rice cakes with 3½ ounces red salmon, sliced tomato, beetroot and unlimited green salad. 3 rockmelon wedges.

* Avocado and salad sandwich on wholegrain bread spread with 1 teaspoon tahini. 1 mandarin.

* Wholemeal roll with 1 sliced boiled egg, lettuce, sprouts, cucumber and 1 teaspoon Kraft Light Mayonnaise. No butter or margarine. Juice or fruit serving.

* Bowl of Zucchini Soup (recipe page 145) with a wholemeal bread roll and small green salad. 1 apple.

* Omelette made from 2 medium eggs with 1 tablespoon low-fat milk or soy milk, 5 halved cherry tomatoes, chopped fresh mushrooms, chopped chives or shallots, 1 dessertspoon chopped parsley, sprinkle of paprika if desired. Small bunch grapes.

* 2 ounces sardines in spring water, drained, 1 tablespoon cottage cheese, sliced tomato and unlimited green salad. 2 Ryvita crackers. Juice or fruit serving.

* ½ pocket bread with 1 tablespoon of Hummus (recipe page 154) or 2 ounces of cottage cheese, salad of your choice, 1 Falafel (recipe page 170). Fruit or juice serving.

* ½ grilled chicken breast with garden salad and Mustard Vinaigrette (recipe page 147), grated fresh beetroot mixed with lemon juice. 2 slices fresh pineapple.

* Mushroom Caps (recipe page 152), 1 small jacket potato with 1 dessertspoon Mock Sour Cream (recipe page 148), garden salad. 2 rockmelon wedges.

* 1 jacket potato with Pesto Sauce (recipe page 150), 1 medium beetroot, garden salad. Juice of fruit serving.

* 1 cup cooked pasta spirals with chopped fresh mushroom, cherry tomatoes, capsicum, snow peas, parsley and pine nuts. Add a little Vinaigrette Dressing (recipe page 148) and mix well. 1 kiwifruit.

* 3½ ounces grilled whitefish, garden salad, small jacket potato topped with 1 dessertspoon Mock Sour Cream (recipe page 148). 1 large piece pawpaw.

EVENING

Select any one of the following choices.

EACH SELECTIION = APPROXIMATELY 450 CAL/1890kJ

* 3½ ounces lean, grilled steak, Chilli Sauce (recipe page 149), 2 scoops sweet potato, ½ cup cauliflower, ½ cup carrots, 2 brocolli florets, 6 snow peas, ½ cup fresh green beans. 1 serve fresh fruit.

* ½ grilled chicken breast topped with fresh lime juice, chopped fresh ginger and tarragon. 1 small jacket potato with 1 dessertspoon Mock Sour Cream recipe page 148). 1 medium-sized cooked beetroot, grated carrot, fresh tomato and a large green salad. 1 serve fresh pawpaw.

* Irish Stew (recipe page 165), green salad, 1 small bunch grapes.

* Creamy Fish Rolls with Dill Sauce (recipe page 162), 1 jacket potato, ½ cup carrots, ½ cup green beans, 2 brocolli florets, 2 brussels sprouts. 1 mandarin.

* Low-Calorie Canelloni (recipe page 174), 1 small corn cob, 2 scoops sweet Potato, ½ cup carrots, unlimited green salad. 1 cup sliced banana, strawberries and passionfruit.

* Large bowl Minestrone Soup (recipe page 145), 1 wholemeal bread roll, 1 jacket Potato, 1 cooked beetroot and unlimited garden salad. 1 serve fresh rockmelon.

* Butternut and Cashew Quiche (recipe page 172), ½ cup steamed cauliflower with Parsley Sauce (recipe page 150), ½ cup steamed carrots, garden salad. 1 cup watermelon balls.

* Cabbage Rolls (recipe page 168), 1 jacket potato, 1 scoop pumpkin, ½ cup Carrots, 6 snow peas, 1/4 cup green beans. 1 serve fresh fruit.

* Grilled Lamb and Fruit Kebabs (recipe page 164), Tomato Salsa (recipe page 151), Spinach and Walnut Salad (recipe page 158), 1 tablespoon Hummus (recipe page 154).

* 1 cup cooked spaghetti with Pesto Sauce (recipe page 150), garden salad with carrot sticks and Vinaigrette Dressing (recipe page 148). 1 pear.

* Baked Fish with Fruit Filling (recipe page 163), 2 scoops sweet potato, 1 medium corn cob, ½ cup cauliflower, 1/4 cup peas, ½ cup green beans. 3 tamarillos.

* Calamari Thai Salad (recipe page 159) with ¾ cup cooked brown rice, Cucumber Salad (recipe page 161). 2 slices pineapple.

LYMPHATIC SHAPE EATING PLAN

Your body type is prone to weight excess but with perseverance you will achieve the most rewarding results. Because of lymphatic congestion you may tire easily, are prone to increased mucus production and swollen gland. If you continue to follow a diet that contains dairy products, salt and processed foods, your obesity will gradually increase over the years.

I have designed an eating plan for you that will stimulate your sluggish metabolism and circulation and improve your liver and kidney function, resulting in more efficient elimination. I will also detoxify your congested lymphatic system.

The best time for you to eat is in the mornings and at lunchtime when your metabolism is most active.

You will enjoy an ample breakfast as this is the best time for your body type and you will remain alert and energetic throughout the morning.

> Lunch is to be your main meal of the day. Your metabolism will cope well with food at this time. Within the sample menus you will find a good selection of protein and carbohydrate foods to keep your blood-sugar levels stable throughout the afternoon.

You must always include raw or steamed green vegetable and salad with your meals to assist digestive processes. For instance, never settle for pasta with a sauce alone, always include a green salad with it. If you are having soup with a wholemeal bread roll, eat some salad vegetables as well.

Your danger period will be late afternoon when you start to feel tired. You may experience false hunger at this time and may be tempted to break your diet. To give in and eat fast food or dairy products (which you will naturally crave) will slow down your progress.

With your body type, even the addition of some cottage cheese is enough to stop changes in body shape and well-being.

Your best snack is raw celery, carrot and apple. I also encourage you to drink fresh vegetable juices. Some good choices are: carrot and celery, carrot and apple, carrot, celery and beetroot, carrot and watermelon. These are great for your kidneys, liver and the elimination of cellulite.

Eat a small meal in the evening when your metabolism is sluggish. You will enjoy a peaceful night's sleep and wake feeling refreshed and much lighter.

LYMPHATIC GUIDELINES

FOOD GROUPS	DESIRABLE FOODS	UNDESIRABLE
Grains, Cereal, Bread and pasta	Wholegrains such as brown rice, corn, rye wheat, buckwheat, oats millet and barley. Bread, crispbread, flour and pasta containing these wholegrains.	Highly refined and bleached white flour products such as white bread, packaged cakes and biscuits. Avoid products made from bakers' flour or breadmaking flour.
Pulses and beans	All beans, lentils and peas. Bean sprouts. Tofu and houmus.	
Meat, chicken, game and fish	Choose lean cuts of red meats and trim off fat before cooking. Free range chickens, turkeys and eggs. Fresh and tinned fish. Shellfish and oysters.	Processed meats, sausages, fried foods. Roast meat dinners. Battery hens and eggs. Skin on poultry Offal meats. Bacon. Anchovies.
Dairy products	None allowed, so substitute with Rice milk low-fat soy milk and soy products. Oat milk, almond milk, Coconut milk.	All dairy products including cream, cheese, butter, icecream, milk, yoghurt and chocolate. Sheep and goats' milk products.
Fruit and vegetables	All fresh and dried fruits, tinned fruit in natural juice. A wide variety of fresh vegetables.	Fruit in sugar syrup. Glacé fruit. Olives

LYMPHATIC GUIDELINES

FOOD GROUPS	DESIRABLE FOODS	UNDESIRABLE
Nuts and Seeds	Unsalted raw nuts and seeds. Tahini and raw nut pastes.	Peanuts and salted nuts. Peanut butter.
Fats and oils	Olive oil. Linseed and canola oil, in moderation only. Tahini, hummus, avocado, nut spreads	Copha, dripping, ghee Butter, suet and lard. Margarine.
Beverages	Water: 8-12 glasses. Mineral and soda water. Cereal beverages. Herb teas. Tannin-free tea. 1-2 cups coffee per day.	Carbonated soft drinks. Mix-up cordials. Malted milk drinks. Alcohol. Tannin-rich tea Chocolate drinks.
Miscellaneous	Very small amounts of honey, sugar or molasses.	Refined sugars and products containing sugars. MSG-621 salt and salty foods Artificial additives, preservatives and colours.

WEIGHT LOSS FOR THE LYMPATHIC BODY SHAPE

On waking have a large glass of water with a squeeze of lemon or lime juice.

BREAKFAST

Select any **one** of the following choices.

EACH SELECTION = APPROXIMATELY 300 CAL/1260kJ

* 1 ounce breakfast cereal (list page 195) with 3½ ounces soy milk or Rice milk. Add 1 dessertspoon oatbran and 1 tablespoon mixed roasted sesame and sunflower seeds, ½ a banana and 3 strawberries.

* 1 cup cooked oats with 3½ ounces Rice milk or soy milk. ½ cup fresh berries and 1 dessertspoon LSA (see page 209).

* 1/4 pawpaw blended with 7 ounces soy milk or Rice milk, ice cubes and 1 heaped teaspoon each of lecithin, wheatgerm and oatbran. 1 slice raisin or fruit loaf.

* 1 slice dry wholemeal toast with ½ medium avocado topped with fresh lime or lemon juice and black pepper. 7 ounces freshly squeezed orange juice.

* 1 poached egg on 1 slice dry wholemeal toast, pour over Blender Hollandaise (recipe page 149) and fresh parsley. Serve with fresh tomato and sprouts. 2 wedges rockmelon.

* ½ cup cooked barley and 5 ounces soy milk, top with 1 tablespoon raisins and 1 dessertspoon LSA (see page 209).

* 1 slice dry wholemeal toast with ½ cup low-salt baked beans sprinkled with fresh parsley and roasted sesame seeds. Serve with fresh tomato and shredded lettuce. ½ small pawpaw.

* 2 slices dry wholemeal toast spread with 1 tablespoon Houmos (recipe page 154). Top with lightly cooked mushroom and crushed garlic served with alfalfa sprouts. ½ cup of sliced kiwifruit and strawberries.

* 2 Wholemeal Pancakes (recipe page 182) with ½ banana, 3 strawberries, pawpaw and passionfruit. Cup of tea.

* 2 Oatbran and Apple Muffins (recipe page 182). 1 apple and 1 orange Cup of tea.

* 1 toasted wholemeal muffin spread thinly with 2 teaspoons tahini and topped with fresh tomato slices, sprouts and freshly ground black pepper. 1 serve fruit or juice.

* 2 slices dry toasted rye bread with 2 ounces sardines in spring water (drained) and finely chopped onion and parsely. Serve with fresh tomato and snow pea sprouts 1 serve fruit or juice.

LUNCH

Select any one of the following choices.

EACH SELECTION = APPROXIMATELY 400 CAL/1680kJ

* Quick Curried Eggs (recipe page 172) with green salad and No Oil Dressing (recipe page 148), 1 slice of dry wholemeal toast. 1 kiwifruit.

* 3½ ounces red salmon (drained). 1 small potato. 1 tablespoon Hummus (recipe page 154), green salad. 1 serve fresh fruit or juice.

* 3½ ounces fresh baked or grilled whitefish, Tomato Salsa (recipe page 151), 1 small potato. Mushroom and Snow Pea Salad (recipe page 159).1 serve fresh fruit or juice.

* 3½ ounces lean grilled steak with Chilli Sauce (recipe page 149), 1 scoop pumpkin, ½ cup carrots, ½ cup green beans and 8 snow peas. 1 serve fresh fruit or juice.

* Open Soy or Lentil Burger (recipe page 170) on wholemeal bread roll with garden salad, sliced beetroot and grated carrot. 1 slice fresh or unsweetened pineapple.

* 1 cup cooked corn pasta spirals with 2 teaspoons Mustard Vinaigrette (recipe page 147), 3½ ounces tuna in spring water (drained) and chopped celery, mushrooms, brocolli, tomato, shallots and artichoke hearts. 2 rockmelon wedges.

* ½ pocket bread filled with 1 Falafel (recipe page 170), 1 tablespoon Hummus (recipe page 154), ½ avocado, green salad. 1 serve fresh Fruit or juice.

* ½ avocado and a mixed salad that includes beetroot and grated carrot on a wholemeal roll. 1 serve fresh fruit or juice.

* ½ grilled chicken breast with Chilli Sauce (recipe page 149) garden salad with fresh lemon juice, 1 small corn cob and 1 jacket potato. 2 slices fresh pineapple.

* 1 cooked cup of spaghetti with Pesto Sauce (recipe page 150) and garden salad with fresh lemon juice. 1 serve fresh fruit or juice.

* Bowl of Minestrone Soup (recipe page 145), 1 wholemeal muffin, Green Vegetable Plate with Dukkah (recipe page 156). 1 serve fresh fruit.

* Lime Chicken Salad (recipe page 160) ¾ cup cooked brown rice. 1 serve Fresh pawpaw.

EVENING

Select any one of the following choices.

EACH SELECTION = APPROXIMATELY 300 CAL/1260kJ

* Calamari Thai Salad (recipe page 159), ½ cup brown rice. ½ cup fresh berries.

* Braised Steak (recipe page 165), green salad. 1 serve fresh fruit.

* Alternative Cannelloni (recipe page 174), green salad with lemon juice. ½ cup mixed sliced kiwifruit, strawberries and passionfruit.

* Creamy Fish Rolls with Dill Sauce (recipe page 162), garden salad with Vinaigrette Dressing (recipe page 148).

* Baked Whole Fish with Fruit Filling (recipe page 163), garden salad with No Oil Dressing (recipe page 148), 1 medium beetroot.

* ½ grilled chicken breast with Pesto Sauce (recipe page 150), garden salad. 1 kiwifruit.

* Quick Mexican Beans (recipe page 171), garden salad with No Oil Dressing (recipe page 148). 1 slice dry rye toast. 2 tamarillos.

* Italian Noodle Soup (recipe page 146), 4 wholemeal Premium crackers, green salad. 1 pear.

* Minestrone Soup (recipe page 145) with 2 slices dry wholemeal toast, Garden salad. 1 serve pawpaw.

* Satay Chicken Kebabs (recipe page 164), ½ cup cooked brown rice, Green salad with raisins and lemon juice.

* 3½ ounces lean grilled steak with Chilli Sauce (recipe page 149), 1 scoop pumpkin, ½ cup carrots, ½ cup green beans, 2 brussell sprouts. 1 slice pineapple.

* Butternut and Cashew Quiche (recipe page 172), garden salad with Lemon juice. 1 nectarine.

Thyroid Shape Eating Plan

Often it is the thyroid type of woman who comes to my clinic for advice because she is too thin and would love to put on some weight. She is often tired, stressed and experiencing mood swings.

The reason for this is the dominance of the thyroid gland, which keeps her metabolic rate so high that she burns calories very quickly.

The positive side to this is that she has less risk of high cholesterol or obesity - provided her diet contains the correct balance of complex carbohydrates and protein.

The negative side is a tendency to continually stimulate her body with caffeine, alcohol, refined carbohydrates, sweets or nicotine. This overstimulates and eventually exhausts the thyroid gland. When this happens she may gain weight very quickly.

If you have become overweight and identify with this body type you should follow the weight loss regime for thyroid shapes, which distributes calories evenly between breakfast, lunch and dinner. All meals are substantial and are designed to regulate energy fluctuations which are so common in thyroid types.

Never skip breakfast and avoid coffee in the mornings or you will be craving stimulants all day

> You must have some protein food at every meal to stimulate your adrenal energy and to moderate your metabolism. Eat lots of wholegrains, cereals, legumes and pulses to maintain stable blood-sugar levels and eliminate mood swings and sweet cravings.

You tolerate dairy products well and the addition of natural low-fat yoghurt with fruit will be more satisfying than eating fruit alone.

Late afternoon is your danger period when energy is at a low ebb. Avoid cake, chocolate or sweets as they will add empty calories and will not be as satisfying.

If you are not overweight and have not exhausted your thyroid gland, then forget the weight loss programme and follow the advice in our maintenance strategy - STEP TWO - to achieve optimum health.

THYROID GUIDELINES

FOOD GROUPS	DESIRABLE FOODS	UNDESIRABLE
Grains, Cereal, Bread And pasta cakes	Wholegrains such as brown rice, corn, rye, wheat, buckwheat, oats millet and barley. Bread, crispbread, flour and pasta containing these wholegrains.	Highly refined and bleached white flour products such as white bread, biscuits and cakes. Avoid products made from breakmaking or baker's flour.
Pulses and Beans	All beans, lentils, and peas. Bean sprouts. Tofu and houmos.	
Meat, chicken, game and fish	Lean red meats. Chicken, turkey and eggs. Fish and Seafood.	Processed meats. Smoked and pickled meats, and smoked seafood.
Dairy products	Most dairy products. Mild cheeses. Sheep and goat's milk and yoghurt. Low-salt fetta cheese.	Strong mature cheeses Chocolate.
Fruit and vegetables	All fresh and dried fruits, tinned fruit in natural juice. A wide variety of fresh vegetables.	Fruit in sugar syrup, glace fruit.
Nuts and seeds	Unsalted raw nuts and seeds. Tahini and raw nut pastes. Peanut Butter. Coconut.	Peanuts and salted nuts.

THYROID GUIDELINES

FOOD GROUPS	DESIRABLE FOODS	UNDESIRABLE
Fats and oils	Linseed, olive and canola oil. coconut	Copha, dripping, ghee suet and lard. Butter.
Beverages	Water 6-12 glasses Mineral and soda water. Cereal beverages. Some herb teas. Tannin-free tea. Decaffeinated coffee.	Carbonated soft drinks, Cola drinks containing Caffeine. Alcohol Tannin-rich coffee. Caffeine-rich coffee. Chocolate drinks.
Miscellaneous	Very small amounts of honey, sugar or molasses.	Refined sugars and products containing sugars. MSG-621. Artificial additives, preservatives and colour. Salt.

STEP ONE

WEIGHT LOSS FOR THE THYROID BODY SHAPE

On waking have a large glass of water with a squeeze of lemon or lime juice.

BREAKFAST

Select any one of the following choices.

EACH SELECTION = APPROXIMATELY 300 CAL 1260kJ

* 1 medium-sized poached egg with Blender Hollandaise (recipe page 149) and freshly chopped parsley, 1 slice wholegrain toast served with fresh tomato and alfalfa or snow pea sprouts. 1 serve fresh fruit or juice.

* ½ cup low-salt baked beans, 1 slice wholemeal toast, fresh tomato slices and alfalfa sprouts. ½ small pawpaw.

* 1 to 2 ounces chopped sardines in spring water (drained) and fresh chopped chives mixed with 1 ounce ricotta cheese served on 2 slices wholegrain toast. 7 ounces freshly squeezed orange juice.

* 2 small eggs beaten with 1 dessertspoon low-fat calcium-enriched milk, mix in 3 chopped cherry tomatoes, mushrooms and fresh dill or coriander. Lightly cook and serve with 1 slice wholegrain toast. 1 serve fruit or juice.

* 1 cup cooked rolled oats and 3½ ounces low-fat calcium-enriched milk, topped with 1 dessertspoon LSA (recipe page 209) and 1 dessertspoon natural yoghurt. ½ cup berries of your choice.

* ½ cup cooked fresh mushrooms served on 1 wholemeal muffin spread with 1 tablespoon Hummus (recipe page 154), top with fresh chopped parsley. 1 serve fresh fruit of your choice.

* 1 ounce breakfast cereal (list page 195), 3½ ounces low-fat calcium

enriched milk or soy milk, add a dessertspoon each of LSA (see page 209) and natural yoghurt, top with sliced banana and strawberries.

* 3½ ounces low-fat natural yoghurt blended with 5 ounces low-fat calcium enriched milk, ice cubes, ¾ cup fresh berries, 1 dessertspoon LSA (see page 209) and 1 dessertspoon wheatgerm. 1 slice raisin or fruit loaf.

* 1 ounce reduced-fat mild cheese grilled on 2 slices wholemeal toast, topped with chopped capsicum, mushroom and chives. 7 ounces fresh orange juice.

* 2 slices rye bread topped with 1/4 avocado, fresh lemon or lime juice, black pepper and sprouts. 2 slices pineapple.

* 2 Wholemeal Pancakes (recipe page 182) with ½ cup mixed sliced banana, strawberries and passionfruit. 1 tablespoon natural yoghurt.

* ½ cup cooked barley with 3½ ounces low-fat calcium-enriched milk,1 tablespoon natural yoghurt, 1 dessertspoon LSA (see page 209), 1½ tablespoons raisins or sultanas, 1 dessertspoon wheatgerm.

LUNCH

Select any **one** of the following choices.

EACH SELECTION = APPROXIMATELY 300 CALORIES/1260kJ

* 2 Ryvita crackers with 1 tablespoon Hummus (recipe page 154), 2 ounces red salmon, sliced tomato, onion, cucumber, sprouts and freshly ground black pepper. 2 wedges rockmelon.

* 1 wholemeal bread roll filled with 1 ounce chicken, Kraft Light Mayonnaise and unlimited salad. ½ cup sliced kiwifruit and strawberries.

* 2 slices rye bread with 1 ounce low-salt fetta cheese, sliced tomato, alfalfa sprouts and freshly ground black pepper. 1/4 fresh pawpaw.

* ½ pocket bread filled with 1 Falafel (recipe page 170), 1 tablespoon Hummus (recipe page 154) and unlimited salad and sprouts. 1 serve fresh fruit or juice.

* Bowl Minestrone soup (recipe page 145), 1 wholemeal muffin, green Salad vegetables. Small bunch of grapes.

* 1 taco filled with Quick Mexican Beans (recipe page 171), shredded lettuce, sliced tomato, alfalfa sprouts and topped with 1 tablespoon natural yoghurt and Chilli Sauce (recipe page 149). 1 serve fresh fruit or juice.

* 1 medium jacket potato with Pesto Sauce (recipe page 150), Mushroom and Snow Pea Salad (recipe page 159). ½ cup fruit salad.

* 3½ ounces grilled fish topped with lemon juice and chopped fennel (if desired), Slimmers' Egg and Potato Salad (recipe page 158), garden salad with No Oil Dressing (recipe page 148). 2 slices fresh pineapple.

* 3 ounces grilled lean meat with Tomato Salsa (recipe page 151), green salad vegetables topped with lemon juice and roasted sesame seeds, 1 slice of rye bread. 1 kiwifruit.

* Calamari Thai Salad (recipe page 159) with ½ cup cooked brown rice.1 cup watermelon balls.

* Greek Salad (recipe page 159), 2 Rye Snacks, 1 mandarin.

* 1 cup pasta of your choice mixed with fresh chopped mushrooms, cherry tomatoes, shallots, capsicum, snow peas and 2 ounces tuna in spring water (drained). You may add a little No Oil Dressing (recipe page 148). 1 wedge rockmelon and 1 wedge honeydew.

EVENING

Select any **one** of the following choices.

EACH SELECTION = APPROXIMATELY 400 CAL/1680kJ

* 3½ ounces lean grilled fillet steak with Blender Hollandaise Sauce (recipe page 149), 2 scoops sweet potato, ½ cup of carrots, 1/4 cup peas, 2 brocolli florets. 2 slices fresh pineapple.

* 3½ ounces lightly grilled veal with Napolitana Sauce (recipe page 175) 1 jacket potato with Mock Sour Cream (recipe page 148), large garden salad with lemon juice. 1 serve fresh fruit.

* Baked Fish with Fruit Filling (recipe page 163), 1 jacket potato with Mock Sour Cream (recipe page 148), green salad with Mustard Vinaigrette (recipe page 147).

* ½ grilled chicken breast with Tomato Salsa (recipe page 151), Slimmers' Egg and Potato Salad (recipe page 158), steamed brocilli, green beans and snow peas. ½ cup sliced banana, strawberry and passionfruit.

* Butternut and Cashew Quiche (recipe page 172), 1 medium beetroot Grated and mixed with a little lemon juice, 1 grated carrot, large garden Salad with Mustard Vinaigrette (recipe page 147). 1 serve fresh fruit.

* Papaya and Chicken Salad (recipe page 161) with 1 cup cooked brown rice.

* Cabbage Rolls (recipe page 168), 1 jacket potato and large garden salad with lemon juice. ½ cup fresh berries.

* Low-Calorie Cannelloni (recipe page 174), 2 scoops sweet potato, ½ cup Carrots, ½ cup cauliflower, 2 brocolli florets. Sprinkle vegetables with Roasted sesame and sunflower seeds. 1 serve fresh fruit.

* 2 Soy Bean and Lentil Patties (recipe page 170), Spinach Salad (recipe page 158), 1 jacket potato. 2 wedges rockmelon

* 1 cup cooked spaghetti with Slimmers' Bolognaise Sauce (recipe page 173),green salad with lemon juice. 1 nectarine.

* Grilled Pork and Pineapple Kebabs (recipe page 164), 2 medium beetroot, Spinach Salad (recipe page 158).

* 3½ ounces grilled fish with parsley sauce (recipe page 150), Green VegetablePlate with Dukkah (recipe page 156), 1 scoop pumpkin, ½ cup carrots.1 serve fresh pawpaw or mango.

MAINTENANCE

CONGRATULATIONS ON YOUR SUCCESS!

You took up the challenge and you made the commitment to lose weight and change your body shape. You made a decision to be healthy and you have achieved the result.

In order to do it, you had to become more active, change your attitude, your eating habits and your cooking methods. Change never comes easily but you found your power and you took control. You made the right choices. YOU did it!

Put the book down for a moment and go take a long look at yourself in the mirror. Look at yourself with pride and know that the person you see is worthy of compliments.

You must never allow anybody or anything to undermine your self-esteem again.

> Remember that your achievements are proof of your inner strength and your ability to do things for yourself.

THE TRANSITION TO WEIGHT MAINTENANCE

Once you have achieved a weight that (a) pleases you and (b) falls within the healthy weight range (see Chapter Three), you are ready to start our Weight Maintenance Programme-**STEP TWO.** Refer to the table on page 34 to estimate your caloric intake to maintain your current desired weight.

Do not start at that caloric level immediately because you are a unique individual and your level for weight maintenance may not perfectly match that in the table. It is only to be used as a general guideline.

To identify **YOUR** ideal level for weight maintenance you must increase your caloric intake gradually. This will ensure that your make a smooth transition between weight loss and weight maintenance.

Begin by increasing your daily caloric intake by 200 cal/840kJ for the first week of maintenance.

This may be achieved simply by adding some extra servings or fruit and complex carbohydrates. For example:

2 additional serves of fruit and an extra serve of bread.

or

2 additional serves of fruit and an extra ½ cup of rice.

or

2 additional serves of fruit and an extra jacket potato.

Gradually increase your daily intake week by week until you stop losing weight and your body weight stabilises.

At this point you will note your ideal weight for your Maintenance level. It is natural for our weight to fluctuate slightly, so add and subtract 4 pounds from this and you now have a comfortable weight range that you will easily stay within.

As soon as you go above your 4 pounds margin then recommence **STEP ONE**-the Body Shaping Diet weight loss programme, until you are back at your ideal weight and then stick to your Maintenance Programme-**STEP TWO.**

SUCCESSFUL WEIGHT MAINTENANCE

Remember that the Body Shaping Diet allowed you to lose your weight gradually, which makes it much easier to maintain. Be confident, you have worked hard to change your metabolism and you have succeeded. You no longer have to put so much energy into controlling your weight.

As a guideline, I have included a range of sample menus for each body shape which are calculated at 1400 cal/5880 kJ each day. You may need to make adjustments to this, according to your ideal caloric level, to achieve successful maintenance. Choose freely from our recipe section which also has some delicious sweets for special occasions.

The increase in calories in **STEP TWO** allows you the freedom to once again look forward to dinner parties or restaurant meals and even have several courses without fear of weight gain. You can relax a little on birthdays and at other celebrations, as long as they are special occasions and not daily occurrences.

Remember, it's what you do 95 per cent of the time that counts.

Never go back to the negative patterns that caused you to be unhealthy and overweight.

To maintain optimum health and achieve successful weight maintenance you should continue your exercise programme. Even though it may have seemed a chore at first, you know that it helped your weight loss, toned your body and increased your fitness level.

By now you will have found a sport or exercise routine that you look forward to and will continue to enjoy.

I recommend that you weigh yourself once a week at the same time of day.
Self-monitoring of your weight will make it easier to maintain.

If you find your weight is creeping back, due to a lapse in routine, return to **STEP ONE** and increase your exercise. Be sure to eliminate any foods that are high in fat or sugar.

If you are feeling a lack of confidence and self control, be sure to remind yourself of your achievements and ability. Contact a reliable friend or a Counsellor if you need help with a difficult situation.

I encourage you to shop wisely and to continue with your new cooking methods. By now your new habits will have become routine. If some of your old habits start creeping back, think about why you changed them and recommit yourself.

Follow your guidelines for your body shape (beginning on page 92), maintain your exercise programme and enjoy good health.

MAINTENANCE FOR THE ANDROID BODY SHAPE

On waking have a large glass of water with a squeeze of lemon or lime juice.

BREAKFAST

Select any **one** of the following choices

EACH SELECTION = APPROXIMATELY 350 CAL/1470kJ

* 1 Wholemeal Pancake (recipe page 182), 1 cup fresh berries, 7 ounces low-fat natural yoghurt, 1 dessertspoon LSA (recipe page 209). Cup of herbal tea.

* 1 ounce breakfast cereal (list page 195) 3½ ounces low-fat calcium-enriched milk, soy milk or Rice milk, ½ tablespoon each of lecithin and LSA (recipe page 209), 6 medium strawberries. 1 slice wholemeal toast with tahini and sprouts.

* 2 slices dry wholemeal toast with ½ cup of cottage cheese, sliced tomato and alfalfa sprouts. 7 ounces freshly squeezed orange juice.

* 1 cup cooked rolled oats with 3 ½ ounces of low-fat calcium-enriched milk, soy milk or Rice milk and sultanas, ½ sliced banana and 3 strawberries, 1 dessertspoon each LSA (recipe page 209) and wheatgerm. Cup of herbal tea.

* 1 Wholemeal Pancake (recipe page 182) with lightly cooked mushrooms,tomato, bean sprouts and fresh dill, gently mixed into ½ cup ricotta cheese.3 wedges rockmelon.

* 2 sliced dry wholemeal with ½ cup salt-reduced baked beans, fresh tomato slices, alfalfa sprouts and fresh parsley. 3 wedges pawpaw and 1 passionfruit.

* ½ cup fresh fruit (your choice) blended with 7 ounces low-fat calcium enriched milk, soy milk or Rice milk, ice cubes and 1 heaped teaspoonful lecithin and wheatgerm. 2 slices raisin or fruit loaf.

* 1 poached or boiled egg with Blender Hollandaise (recipe page 149) and fresh parsley on 2 slices dry wholemeal toast. Serve with sliced tomato, sprouts and ground black pepper. 7 ounces fresh orange juice.

* 2 Banana and Pecan Muffins (recipe page 183). Cup dandelion beverage.

* 2 slices wholemeal toast spread with Houmos (recipe page 154) top with 2 ounces chopped sardines in spring water (drained) and freshly chopped chives and parsley. 1 serve fresh pawpaw.

* 1 toasted wholemeal muffin topped with Mushroom Sauce (recipe page 150), fresh parsley and roasted sesame seeds. Fresh fruit of your choice.

* 2 slices dry wholemeal toast with ½ avocado, fresh tomato slices, chopped chives and freshly ground black pepper.

LUNCH

Select any **one** of the following choices.

EACH SELECTION = APPROXIMATELY 450 CAL/1890kJ

* Guacamole (recipe page 153), mixed fresh raw vegetables to dip e.g. radish, Fennel, carrot, zucchini, capsicum, celery and broccoli florets. 1 slice Pumpernickel with Hummus (recipe page 154). 1 serve fresh fruit

* 1 pocket bread with 2 Falafel (recipe page 170), lettuce, 1 tablespoon Hummus and Tabbouli (recipe page 155). 1 banana.

* Wholemeal bread roll with a Soy Bean Pattie (recipe page 170), fresh green Salad, tomato, raw grated beetroot and ½ medium avocado. 7 ounces orange juice.

* Bowl of Italian Noodle Soup (recipe page 146), green salad with No Oil Dressing (recipe page 148). 2 slices wholemeal bread. 1 serve rockmelon.

* 4 ounces red salmon and ½ cup cottage cheese, garden salad, 1 medium beetroot. 2 Vita wheat crackers. 1 nectarine.

* 2 slices dry wholemeal toast with 1/3 cup ricotta cheese and 2 ounces drained chopped sardines, fresh tomato slices, onion and fresh parsley. 3 slices fresh pineapple.

* 1 cup cooked corn pasta spirals mixed with 2½ ounces chopped cooked chicken, 4 chopped sun-dried tomatoes, 1 teaspoon olive oil, 3 teaspoons pine nuts and chopped raw mushrooms, shallots, celery, radish, fennel, broccoli, bean sprouts, fresh parsley and mint if desired. 2 tamarillos.

* Mixed Bean and Rice Salad (recipe page 156). 1 nashi fruit.

* Quick Curried Eggs (recipe page 172), garden salad, 1 slice rye bread with Hanini. 6 strawberries.

* Asparagus vinaigrette (recipe page 155), 1 jacket potato with Mock Sour Cream (recipe page 148), 1 medium corn cob, 2 Sesame Ryvita, 4 lychees or rambutans.

* Low-Calorie Cannelloni (recipe page 174), Beetroot and Watercress Salad (recipe page 157), 3 button squash, 1 corn cob. 1 slice rye bread. 1 serve fresh fruit or juice.

* Bowl of Pumpkin soup (recipe page 146), 2 slices rye bread. Spinach and Walnut Salad (recipe page 158). 1 cup watermelon balls.

EVENING

Select any one of the following choices.

EACH SELECTION = APPROXIMATELY 600 CAL/2520kJ

* 3½ ounces grilled white fish with Florentine Sauce (recipe page 150), Tomato Salsa (recipe page 151), 1 jacket potato with 1 dessertspoon of Mock Sour Cream (recipe page 148), 2 scoops sweet potato, 1 medium corn cob, ½ cup green beans, 3 brussel sprouts. ½ cup fruit salad.

* Tuna Bake (recipe page 179), 1 medium beetroot, green salad. 1 serve fresh fruit.

* Green Vegetable Plate with Dukkah (recipe page 156), 1 serve Dahl (recipe page 171), 1 cup cooked brown rice. Banana Cream (recipe page 183) with strawberries and passionfriut.

* 2 small taco shells filled with Quick Mexican Bean Mix (recipe page 171), fresh chopped tomato, shredded lettuce, alfalfa sprouts, low-fat natural yoghurt and Chilli Sauce (recipe page 149). 2 small corn cobs. Lemon Self-Saucing Pudding (recipe page 186).

* 1 bowl Pumpkin Soup (recipe page 146), Open Soy or Lentil Burger (recipe page 170) on a wholemeal bread roll with avocado, salad and sprouts, Chilli Sauce (recipe page 149). 2 slices fresh pineapple.

* Braised Steak (recipe page 165), 1 cup cooked brown rice, garden salad with dressing of your choice. Fresh Fruit Sorbet (recipe page 186).

* 1 bowl Minestrone Soup (recipe page 145), Cannelloni with Sprout Filling (recipe page 174), 2 scoops sweet potato, ½ cup carrots, ½ cup cauliflower, 1/4 cup green peas, ½ cup lightly cooked mushrooms. 1 serve fresh fruit.

* Baked fish with Fruit Filling (recipe page 163), dry baked potato with Mock Sour cream (recipe page 148), Stuffed Mushroom Caps (recipe page 152), 1 cob corn, ½ cup cabbage, ½ cup beans. 1 slice rye bread.

* 2 cups cooked spaghetti with Quick Pesto Sauce (recipe page 150), garden salad with No Oil Dressing (recipe page 148). Fresh pawpaw with passionfruit and strawberries.

* Avocado and Chicken in Filo (recipe page 168), 2 scoops potato mashed With finely chopped onion and parsley, 2 scoops sweet potato, ½ cup Carrots, ½ cup cabbage, 2 brussel sprouts. 1 serve fresh fruit.

* Borlotti Bean Bake (recipe page 169) 1 small jacket potato, Carrot and Sultana Salad (recipe page 158), green Vegetable Plate with Dukkah (recipe page 156). 1 serve fresh fruit.

* Zucchini Soup (recipe page 145) and 2 slices of toasted rye bread. Cabbage Rolls (recipe page 168), 2 scoops sweet potato, ½ cup carrots, 1/4 cup peas and 1/4 cup green beans. Fresh Fruit Sorbet (recipe page 186).

MAINTENANCE FOR THE GYNAEOID BODY SHAPE

On waking have a large glass of water with a squeeze of lemon or lime juice.

BREAKFAST

Select any **one** of the following choices.

EACH SELECTION = APPROXIMATELY 350 CAL/1470kJ

* 1 cup cooked brown rice, 3½ ounces low-fat calcium-enriched milk or soy milk, 1 dessertspoon wheatgerm, ½ banana and 6 small or 3 large strawberries.

* 1 cup cooked rolled oats, 3½ ounces low-fat calcium-enriched milk, skim milk, or low-fat soy milk, sprinkle with roasted sesame and sunflower seeds,1 small banana. 1 slice raisin toast. Cup of herbal tea.

* 1 poached or boiled egg with Blender Hollandaise (recipe page 149) and fresh parsley, 2 slices wholegrain toast, serve with tomato and snow pea sprouts. 7 ounces fresh orange juice.

* Fruit shake: your choice of fruit blended with 8 ounces low-fat calcium enriched milk or soy milk, ice cubes and 1 heaped teaspoon each of LSA (recipe page 209) and wheatgerm. 2 slices raisin or fruit loaf.

* 2 slices wholegrain toast topped with ½ an avocado, squeeze over lemon or lime juice and freshly ground black pepper. Cup of herbal tea.

* 1 ounce breakfast cereal (see list page 195), 3½ ounces low-fat calcium enriched milk or soy milk, 1 dessertspoon wheatgerm, ½ cup fresh berries. 1 slice rye toast with tahini. Cup of dandelion beverage.

* 2 Wholemeal Pancakes (recipe page 182) with sliced banana, passionfruit and pawpaw and Vanilla Yoghurt Sauce (recipe page 190). Cup of herbal tea.

* 2 slices wholemeal toast spread with 1 tablespoon Hummus (recipe page 154), top with 2 ounces sardines in spring water (drained), sliced tomato and parsley. 7 ounces glass freshly squeezed orange juice.

* 1 boiled egg with 1 slice rye toast, 2 Blueberry Muffins (recipe page 183). Cup of tea.

* 1 toasted wholemeal muffin topped with 1/4 cup ricotta cheese, fresh tomato, parsley and freshly ground black pepper. 1 serve fresh paw-paw.

* 2 slices wholemeal toast, ½ cup of salt-reduced baked beans, tomato slices and shredded lettuce. 3 rockmelon wedges.

* 1 toasted wholemeal muffin with Mushroom Sauce (recipe page 150), sprinkle with roasted sesame seeds and fresh parsley. 1 serve fresh fruit or juice.

LUNCH

Select any **one** of the following choices.

EACH SELECTION = APPROXIMATELY 450 CAL/1890kJ

* 3 ½ ounces red salmon, 2 halves devilled Eggs (recipe page 153), sliced tomato, beetroot and unlimited green salad. 1 slice rye bread. 3 slices fresh pineapple.

* Avocado and salad sandwich on wholegrain bread thinly spread with tahini. 7 ounce carton low-fat fruit yoghurt.

* Wholemeal roll with 1 sliced boiled egg, lettuce, sprouts, cucumber and 1 teaspoon Kraft Light Mayonnaise. 1 Apple and Oatbran Muffin (recipe page 182). 1 mandarin.

* Pumpkin Soup (recipe page 146), 1 wholemeal bread roll, garden salad with dressing of your choice. 1 banana.

* Omelette made from 2 eggs and 1 tablespoon low-fat milk, 5 cherry tomatoes, chopped fresh mushroom, chives or shallots and parsley, paprika if desired. 2 slices toast. 1 pear.

* 2 ounces sardines in spring water (drained), 1/4 cup cottage cheese, garden salad with dressing of your choice. 1 wholemeal bread roll. 7 ounces fresh orange juice.

* 1 pocket bread with 2 Falafel (recipe page 170), lettuce, 1 tablespoon Hummus (recipe page 154) and Tabbouli (recipe page 155). 1 banana.

* ½ grilled chicken breast with Florentine Sauce (recipe page 150), garden salad with Mustard Vinaigrette (recipe page 147), grated fresh beetroot mixed with lemon juice. 2 slices fresh pineapple.

* 3½ ounces grilled fish with Blender Hollandaise (recipe page 149) and fresh parsley, Mushroom Caps (recipe page 152), 1 small jacket potato with 1 dessertspoon of Mock Sour Cream (recipe page 148), garden salad. 2 rockmelon wedges.

* Pork and Pineapple Kebabs (recipe page 164), 1 medium beetroot, 1 medium corn cob, Green Bean and Apple Salad (recipe page 157). 1 slice rye bread.

* 1 cup cooked pasta with Pesto Sauce (recipe page 150), garden salad withVinaigrette Dressing (recipe page 148), Carrot and Sultana Salad (recipe Page 158). 1 kiwifruit.

* Mixed Bean and Rice Salad (recipe page 156), 1 large piece pawpaw.

EVENING

Select any one of the following choices.
EACH SELECTION = APPROXIMATELY 600 CAL/2520kJ

* 3½ ounces lean grilled steak, Tomato Salsa (recipe page 151), 2 scoops sweet potato, ½ cup cauliflower, 1 medium corn cob, 3 broccoli florets, 1/4 cup peas, ½ cup fresh green beans. Minted Pineapple Sorbet (recipe page 184).

* ½ grilled chicken breast topped with fresh lime juice, chopped fresh ginger and tarragon. 1 medium jacket potato with 1 dessertspoon Mock Sour Cream (recipe page 148). 1 medium-sized cooked beetroot, Spinach and Walnut Salad (recipe page 158), 1 wedge pawpaw. Iced Mango Treat (recipe page 184).

* Irish Stew (recipe page 165), 2 slices wholemeal toast. ½ custard apple.

* Tandoori Fish (recipe page 162), 1 cup cooked brown rice, Minted Tomato Salsa (recipe page 151), ½ cup green beans, 3 broccoli florets, 3 brussel sprouts. Your choice of 1 cup of mixed fresh fruit.

* Minestrone Soup (recipe page 145) with 1 slice rye bread. Low-Calorie Canelloni (recipe page 174), 1 small corn cob, 2 scoops sweet potato, ½ cup carrots and unlimited green salad with dressing of your choice. 1 serve fresh fruit.

* Chicken and Vegetable Hotpot (recipe page 166) with 1 wholemeal dinner roll, Beetroot and Watercress Salad (recipe page 157). Passionfruit and Rockmelon Mousse (Recipe page 185).

* Butternut and Cashew Quiche (recipe page 172), Greek Salad (recipe page 159). 1 cup fruit salad.

* Cabbage Rolls (recipe page 168), 1 jacket potato, 2 scoops sweet potato, ½ cup carrots, 1/4 cup peas, ½ cup green beans. Minted Pineapple sorbet (recipe page 184).

* Grilled Lamb and Fruit Kebabs (recipe page 164), 1 jacket potato with Mock Sour Cream Dressing (recipe page 148), Tomato Salsa (recipe page 151), Spinach and Walnut Salad (recipe page 158), 1 tablespoon Hummus (recipe page 154).

* 2 cups cooked spaghetti with Pesto Sauce (recipe page 150), garden salad with carrot sticks and Vinaigrette Dressing (recipe page 148). Poached Pears with Almond Custard Cream (recipe page 188).

* Baked Fish with Fruit filling (recipe page 163), 2 scoops sweet potato,1 medium corn cob, ½ cup cauliflower, 1/4 cup peas, ½ cup green beans. Berry Delicious (recipe page 184).

* Chicken in a Parcel (recipe page 179), Pasta Salad (recipe page 157). 1 serve fresh fruit of your choice.

MAINTENANCE FOR THE LYMPHATIC BODY SHAPE

On waking have a large glass of water with a squeeze of lemon or lime juice.

BREAKFAST

Select any **one** of the following choices.

EACH SELECTION = APPROXIMATELY 450 CAL/1890kJ

* 1 ounces breakfast cereal (list page 195) with 3½ ounces soy milk or Rice milk, 1 dessertspoon of oatbran and 1 tablespoon mixed roasted sesame and sunflower seeds. 2 flapjacks (recipe page 189), ½ banana and passionfruit.

* 1 cup cooked oats with 3½ ounces rice milk or soy milk, ½ cup fresh berries and 1 dessertspoon LSA (see page 209). 1 slice wholemeal toast with tahini, tomato and fresh parsley.

* 1/4 pawpaw blended with 7 ounces soy milk or Rice milk, ice cubes and 1 heaped teaspoon each of lecithin, wheatgerm and oatbran. 1 Apple and Oatbran Muffin (recipe page 182). Cup of herbal tea.

* 2 slices dry wholemeal toast with ½ medium-sized avocado topped with fresh lime or lemon juice and black pepper. 7 ounces freshly squeezed orange juice.

* 2 poached eggs, 2 slices dry wholemeal toast, pour over Blender Hollandaise (recipe page 149) and serve with fresh parsley, tomato and sprouts. 1 serve rockmelon.

* 1 cup cooked barley and 5 ounces soy milk, top with 1 tablespoon raisins, 1 dessertspoon LSA (recipe page 209) and 6 strawberries.

* 2 slices dry wholemeal toast with ½ cup low-salt baked beans sprinkled with fresh parsley and roasted sesame seeds, serve with tomato, avocado slices and shredded lettuce. 1/4 pawpaw.

* 2 slices dry wholemeal toast, top with Mushroom Sauce (recipe page 150) and parsley, serve with tomato, sliced avocado and alfalfa sprouts. ½ custard apple.

* 3 Wholemeal Pancakes (recipe page 182) with 1 banana, strawberries, pawpaw and passionfruit. Cup of herbal tea.

* 7 ounces glass soy milk, 2 Oatbran and Apple Muffins (recipe page 182). Cup of herbal tea.

* 1 toasted wholemeal muffin topped with Dahl (recipe page 171) and fresh parsley. 1 serve fruit or juice.

* 2 slices dry toasted rye bread with 3.5 ounces sardines in spring water (drained), finely chopped onion and parsley, serve with fresh tomato and snow pea sprouts. 7 ounces apple juice.

LUNCH

Select any **one** of the following choices.

EACH SELECTION = APPROXIMATELY 550 CAL/2310kJ

* Quick Curried Eggs (recipe page 172), garden salad and No Oil Dressing (recipe page 148), 2 slices of dry wholemeal toast. 1 apple.

* 3½ ounces red salmon (drained), 1 medium potato, ½ cup corn kernels, 1 medium beetroot, garden salad with Hazelnut Dressing (recipe page 148). 2 slices fresh pineapple and 1 kiwifruit.

* 3½ ounces fresh baked or grilled whitefish with Pesto Sauce (recipe page 150), Tomato Salsa (recipe page 151), 1 medium potato, Mushroom and Snow Pea Salad (recipe page 159), 1 slice rye bread. 1 serve fresh pawpaw.

* 3½ ounces lean grilled steak with Mustard Sauce (recipe page 150), 2 scoops pumpkin, ½ cup carrots, ½ cup green beans, 4 brussels sprouts and 8 snow peas. Iced Mango Treat (recipe page 184).

* Open Soy or Lentil Burger (recipe page 170) on wholemeal breadroll with avocado, garden salad, sliced beetroot, grated carrot, fresh pineapple and Chilli Sauce (recipe page 149). 1 serve of fresh fruit or juice of your choice.

* Tuna Bake (recipe page 179), green salad. 2 rockmelon wedges.

* 1 pocket bread filled with 2 Falafel (recipe page 170), 1 tablespoon Hummus (recipe page 154), ½ avocado, garden salad with lemon juice. 7 ounces fresh orange juice.

* Mixed Bean and Rice Salad (recipe page 156). 1 slice pumpernickel with Tahini. 1 serve fresh fruit or juice.

* ½ grilled chicken breast with Chilli Sauce (recipe page 149), garden salad with fresh lemon juice, 1 small corn cob and 1 jacket potato. Baked Rice Pudding (recipe page 185) with banana and passionfruit.

* 2 cups cooked spaghetti with Pesto Sauce (recipe page 150) and garden salad with fresh lemon juice. 1 guava.

* Italian Noodle Soup (recipe page 146), 1 wholemeal muffin, 1 medium corn cob, Green Vegetable Plate with Dukkah (recipe page 156). 1 serve fresh fruit of your choice.

* Papaya and Chicken Salad (recipe page 161), 1 cup cooked brown rice, Cucumber Salad (recipe page 161). 1 serve pawpaw.

EVENING

Select any **one** of the following choices.

EACH SELECTION = APPROXIMATELY 400 CAL/1680kJ

* Calamari Thai Salad (recipe page 159) with 1 cup cooked brown rice. 1 cup fresh berries.

* Braised Steak (recipe page 165), 1 medium corn cob, garden salad with Vinaigrette Dressing (recipe page 148). Fresh Fruit Sorbet (recipe page 186).

* Alternative Cannelloni (recipe page 174), 2 scoops sweet potato, ½ cup Carrots, 3 button squash, ½ cup green beans, 3 broccoli florets. Sliced Kiwifruit, strawberries and passionfruit (mixed).

* Slimmers' Spaghetti Bolognaise (recipe page 173) with 1 cup cooked pasta, garden salad with lemon juice. 6 strawberries.

* Baked Whole Fish with Fruit Filling (recipe page 163), 1 jacket potato, garden salad with No Oil Dressing (recipe page 148), 1 medium beetroot.

* ½ grilled chicken breast with Pesto Sauce (recipe page 150), Tomato Salsa (recipe page 151), 1 medium corn cob, 3 broccoli florets, ½ cup green beans. 1 fruit serve of your choice.

* Quick Mexican Beans (recipe page 171), garden salad with No Oil Dressing (recipe page 148). Babaganouj (recipe page 154) 1 tablespoon Hummus (recipe page 154), ½ pita bread. 1 cup watermelon balls.

* Italian Noodle Soup (recipe page 146), 2 slices toasted rye bread, Beetroot and Watercress Salad (recipe page 157). Poached Pears (recipe page 188).

* Lime Chicken Salad (recipe page 160) with 1 cup cooked brown rice. 1 Serve fresh fruit of your choice.

* Grilled Pork and Pineapple Kebabs (recipe page 164), 1 medium corn Cob, Tabbouli Salad (recipe page 155) Beetroot and Watercress Salad (recipe page 157).

* 3.5 ounces lean grilled steak with Chilli Sauce (recipe page 149), 1 medium corn cob, 1 scoop pumpkin, ½ cup carrots, ½ cup green beans, 2 brussels sprouts. Fresh Fruit Sorbet (recipe page 186).

* Butternut and Cashew Quiche (recipe page 172), Green Bean and Apple Salad (recipe page 157), 1 jacket potato.

STEP TWO

MAINTENANCE FOR THE THYROID BODY SHAPE

On waking have a large glass of water with a squeeze of lemon or lime juice.

BREAKFAST

Select any one of the following choices.

EACH SELECTION = APPROXIMATELY 4OO CAL/1680kJ

* 2 poached eggs with blender Hollandaise (recipe page 149) and freshly chopped parsley, 2 slices of wholegrain toast served with fresh tomato and alfalfa or snow pea sprouts. 7 ounces orange juice.

* ½ cup low-salt baked beans, 2 slices rye toast, bean sprouts, tomato and a little sliced avocado. 2 wedges pawpaw.

* 2 slices wholegrain toast spread with ricotta cheese and topped with 2 ounces sardines in spring water (drained), fresh chives, parsley and freshly ground black pepper, serve with tamarillo cut in halves, sprouts and 1/4 avocado.

* 2 large eggs beaten with a little low-fat calcium-enriched milk, mix in 3 chopped cherry tomatoes and chopped mushrooms and fresh dill or coriander, lightly cook and serve with 2 slices of wholegrain toast. 1 serve fruit or juice of your choice.

* 1 cup cooked rolled oats, 3½ ounces low-fat calcium-enriched milk, top with 1 dessertspoon LSA (recipe page 209) and 1 dessertspoon natural yoghurt, ½ banana and some fresh strawberries. 1 Blueberry Muffin (recipe page 183). Cup of herbal tea.

* ½ cup cooked fresh mushrooms served on 1 wholemeal muffin spread with 1 tablespoon Hummus (recipe page 154), top with fresh chopped parsley. 7 ounces low-fat calcium-enriched milk blended with 1 small banana and flavoured with vanilla and ground nutmeg.

* 1 ounce breakfast cereal (list page 195), 3½ ounces low-fat calcium-enriched milk or soy milk, add a dessertspoon each of LSA (see page 209) and natural yoghurt, top with fresh slices of strawberries and banana. 1 slice wholemeal toast with tahini. Cup of tea.

* 3½ ounces low-fat natural yoghurt blended with 5 ounces low-fat calcium-enriched milk, ice cubes, 1 cup fresh berries, 1 dessertspoon LSA (see page 209) and 1 dessertspoon wheatgerm. 1 Banana and Pecan Muffin (recipe page 183).

* 1 ounce reduced-fat mild cheese grilled on 2 slices of wholemeal toast, top with chopped capsicum, mushroom and chives. 7 ounces fresh orange juice. Fresh papaya.

* 2 slices rye toast with ½ avocado, fresh lemon juice, black pepper and sprouts. 1 pear. 7 ounce glass of low-fat calcium-enriched milk.

* 2 Wholemeal Pancakes (recipe page 183) with 1 sliced banana, strawberries and passionfruit, Vanilla Yoghurt Sauce (recipe page 190).

* 1 cup cooked barley with 3½ ounces low-fat calcium-enriched milk, 1 tablespoon natural yoghurt, 1 dessertspoon LSA (see page 209), 1½ tablespoons raisins or sultanas, 1 dessertspoon wheatgerm.

LUNCH

Select any **one** of the following choices.

EACH SELECTION = APPROXIMATELY 450 CAL/1890 kJ

* 2 slices rye toast with 1 tablespoon Hummus (recipe page 154), 3½ ounces red salmon, sliced tomato, onion, cucumber, sprouts and freshly ground black pepper. 2 wedges rockmelon.

* 1 wholemeal bread roll filled with 2 ounces chicken, Kraft Light Mayonnaise, ½ avocado and unlimited salad. ½ cup sliced kiwifruit and strawberries.

* Greek Salad (recipe page 159), Babaganouj (recipe page 154), ½ Pita bread. 1/4 pawpaw.

* 1 pocket bread with 2 Falafel (recipe page 170), 1 tablespoon Hummus (recipe page 154) and Tabbouli Salad (recipe page 155) lettuce and sprouts. 1 serve fresh fruit or juice.

* Italian Noodle Soup (recipe page 146), 1 wholemeal muffin, Fresh Asparagus vinaigrette (recipe page 155). Small bunch of grapes.

* 2 tacos filled with Quick Mexican Beans (recipe page 171), grated low fat cheese, shredded lettuce, sliced tomato, alfalfa sprouts and topped with natural yoghurt and Chilli Sauce (recipe page 149). 1 serve fresh fruit or juice.

* Chickpea Curry (recipe page 178), ½ cup brown rice, Beetroot and Watercress Salad (recipe page 157). ½ cup fruit salad.

* 3½ ounces grilled fish topped with Egg Sauce (recipe page 150), garden salad with No Oil Dressing (recipe page 148), Carrot and Sultana Salad (recipe page 158). 2 slices fresh pineapple.

* 3½ ounces grilled lean meat with Tomato Salsa (recipe page 151), 1 jacket potato with Mock Sour Cream (recipe page 148), green salad vegetables topped with lemon juice and roasted sesame seeds, 1 slice of rye bread. 1 kiwifruit.

* Calamari Thai Salad (recipe page 159) with 1 cup cooked brown rice. Cucumber Salad (recipe page 161). ½ custard apple.

* Salmon Mornay (recipe page 180), green salad with lemon juice. Fresh fruit of your choice.

* Mixed Bean and Rice Salad (recipe page 156). Mixed rockmelon, water Melon and honeydew balls.

EVENING

Select any **one** of the following choices.

EACH SELECTION = APPROXIMATELY 550 CAL/2310kJ

* 1 cup cooked pasta with Eggplant and Napolitana Sauce (recipe page 175). 1 serve fresh pineapple and strawberries.

* Caribbean Chicken (recipe page 178), ½ cup cooked rice, Green Vegetable Plate with Dukkah (recipe page 156). Fresh Fruit Sorbet (recipe page 186).

* Tuna Bake (recipe page 179), green salad. Fresh fruit of your choice.

* Chicken in a Parcel (recipe page 179), Slimmers' Egg and Potato Salad (recipe page 158), steamed broccoli, green beans and snow peas. ½ cup sliced kiwifruit and strawberries.

* Butternut and Cashew Quiche (recipe page 172), 1 medium beetroot Grated and mixed with a little lemon juice, 1 grated carrot, 1/4 avocado, 1 cob corn, garden salad with Mustard Vinaigrette (recipe page 147). 1 cup melon balls.

* Seafood Salad (recipe page 160) with ¾ cup of cooked brown rice. Berry Delicious (recipe page 184).

* Cabbage Rolls (recipe page 168), 1 jacket potato, large garden salad with lemon juice. Apple Crumble (recipe page 187) with Almond Custard Cream (see recipe page 188).

* Irish Stew (recipe page 165), ½ cup brown rice, green salad. Fresh fruit Sorbet (recipe page 186).

* 2 Soy Bean or Lentil Patties (recipe page 170), 1 jacket potato with Pesto Sauce (recipe page 150), 1 medium corn cob, Spinach and Walnut Salad (recipe page 158). Small bunch grapes.

* 1 cup cooked spaghetti with Authentic Bolognaise Sauce (recipe page 180), green salad with lemon juice. Fresh Fruit Sorbet (recipe page 186).

* Lamb and Fruit Kebabs (recipe page 164), ½ cup cooked brown rice, 1 medium beetroot, 1 medium corn cob, Spinach Salad (recipe page 158).

* 3½ ounces grilled fish with Parsley Sauce (recipe page 150), Green Vegetable Plate with Dukkah (recipe page 156), 2 scoops pumpkin, ½ cup carrots. Minted Pineapple Sorbet (recipe page 184).

BODY TYPE WEIGHT CONTROL SUPPLEMENTS

These supplements are tailor-made for your body type and are scientifically designed by Dr. Sandra Cabot

Each of the 4 Body Types has unique hormonal & metabolic characteristics. That's why some people put on weight easily and others don't! Balance your metabolism for your body type.

LYMPHATIC WEIGHT CONTROL TABLETS

These are known as "L - Body Type Figure Control" Tablets
Each tablet contains –
Fenugreek 200 mg
Rutin 50 mg
Selenomethionine 4 mcg
Celery 12.5 mg
Horseradish 12.5 mg
Fennel 12.5 mg
Kelp 25mg
Cayenne fruit powder 2.5 mg
Vitamin B 6 – 2.5 mg

Lymphatic women benefit from this combination because it can —
Boost their sluggish metabolic rate
Relieve fluid retention
Eliminate mucus & toxins
Improve the lymphatic system

These actions will increase their ability to burn fat and eliminate excess fluid. Weight loss will then occur from all over the body and particularly the swollen areas of the limbs and cellulite areas. It then becomes possible for them to lose weight easily and their bone structure will become much more obvious. For the first time in their lives they will find it easy to lose weight which is a great relief because they have often been over weight since childhood. An extra benefit is that their general health will improve giving them more energy and making them less likely to suffer with infections and allergies.

Extra points for Lymphatic women –
They must avoid ALL DAIRY PRODUCTS (milk, butter, cheese, yoghurt, icecream, cream & chocolate) & margarine
They must drink plenty of pure water
They need to exercise regularly to aid their lymphatic system
They benefit from spicy foods (eg. curries, chilli, turmeric, coriander, garlic & ginger etc.)

GYNAEOID WEIGHT CONTROL TABLETS

These are known as "G – Body Type Figure Control" Tablets
Each tablet contains –
Wild Yam 150 mg
Parsley Piert 25 mg
Vitex Agnes Castus 50mg
Gymnema Sylvestre 25mg
Chromium picolinate 67 mcg

Gynaeoid women benefit from this combination because it can --
Increase natural progesterone production in the body
Reduce estrogen dominance
Reduce cravings for sweet creamy foods
Reduce cellulite in the buttocks & thighs
Reduce fluid retention in the buttocks & thighs
These actions will reduce the effect of estrogen on the buttocks & thighs enabling weight loss from these areas. Fat will be metabolised & converted into muscle.
Weight loss will occur from the buttocks & thighs & not from the face & breasts. Hormonal problems such as heavy bleeding, fibroids & PMT will reduce. Cravings for foods combining fat & sugars together will reduce.

Extra points for Gynaeoid women --

They must avoid foods combining fat & sugar together (eg. chocolate, cream cakes, sweet biscuits, custards and icecream)
They should have regular protein such as fish, eggs, seafood, free range chicken (without the skin), nuts, seeds & legumes & wholemeal cereals & bread.
They should exercise the legs & buttocks with an exercise bike, brisk walking, skipping & swimming.

ANDROID WEIGHT CONTROL TABLETS
These are known as "A – Body Type Figure Control" Tablets
Each tablet contains -
Chitosan 250 mg
Milk Thistle 25mg
Red Clover 25mg
Hops 25 mg
Dong Quai 25 mg
Choline 12.5mg
Inositol 12.5mg

Android women benefit from this combination because it can --
Balance their hormones so that excess levels of male hormones (androgens) are reduced, and the levels of female hormones (estrogen and progesterone) are maintained. This will make the figure line more feminine and increases weight loss from the abdomen and trunk. This will also help to reduce the signs of excessive male hormones such as acne, facial and body hair and scalp hair loss.

Hops is probably the most estrogenic of all the herbs and its female effect can be augmented with Red Clover and Dong Quai.

Improve their liver function so that the ability of the liver to burn fat increases. This will reduce abdominal obesity and restore the waistline. Other benefits of improved liver function are lowered cholesterol levels and improvement of blood sugar metabolism. Type II diabetes can be reduced, or in many cases reversed completely with improved liver function and weight loss. Milk Thistle, Choline and Inositol are beneficial lipotrophic factors for the liver.

Android women can benefit from natural fiber such as chitosan, which reduces the absorption of saturated fat from the foods in the diet. This will reduce the amount of fat returning back to the liver from the gut after eating. Chitosan is a proven substance for reducing the absorption of fat.

Extra points for Android women –
They must reduce their intake of saturated fats and salt. The foods that should be avoided are full cream dairy products, cheese, butter, cream, icecream, chocolate, deep fried foods, fatty meats, preserved meats (ham, pizza meats, bacon, sausage, delicatessen meats, smoked meats) and animal skins. Alcohol intake should be reduced.

Android women need to eat plenty of salads & fruit as the liver function is improved by eating these raw living foods. Raw vegetable juices are excellent and can be taken with a liver tonic powder such as Livatone Plus.

Protein can be derived from all types of seafood, eggs (boiled or poached), lean red meats and by combining grains, nuts, seeds & legumes. Generally speaking protein is good for androids as it reduces blood sugar levels and improves insulin resistance.

Android women are usually strong and muscular and benefit from aerobic exercise such as swimming, brisk walking and aerobic workouts.

THYROID WEIGHT CONTROL TABLETS

These are known as "T – Body Type Figure Control" Tablets
Each tablet contains -
Chromium picolinate 67 mcg
Glutamine 100 mg
Liquorice 75 mg
Ginseng 75 mg
Magnesium chelate 200 mg
Zinc chelate 2 mg
Vitamin B 5 -- 10 mg

Thyroid women benefit from this combination because it can --

Improve the function of their adrenal glands thus producing increased and sustained energy levels. Reduce cravings for stimulants and sugary foods, which will make it much easier to follow a healthy eating program. Reduce the lows in blood sugar levels and energy so typical of this body type.
Increase the conversion of fat into muscle.
Reduce stress levels.

Extra Points for Thyroid women ---

They should avoid artificial sweeteners, synthetic diet pills, and smoking and excess levels of caffeine.
They should avoid refined sugars found in white flour & white sugar.
They will benefit from herbal teas containing dandelion, chamomile & peppermint and dandelion coffee.
Thyroid women need to eat regular meals containing complex carbohydrates (cereals, wholemeal breads, grains, nuts, seeds, legumes, wholemeal pasta etc.) and protein from seafood, eggs, lean red meats, free range chicken & legumes.
Thyroid women need to do regular exercise to build up their bone density and increase muscle mass. Suitable exercises are brisk walking (with hand weights), aerobic workouts, sports, swimming and weight training.

<u>Dosage</u> of the Body Type supplements is: one tablet three times daily just before food
Drink 8 glasses of pure water daily & increase fiber in the diet.

This is your "weight loss lifeline" dedicated to all those people who seriously want to control their weight.

Carrying excess weight not only slows down your every step but also slows down all the major organs in your body. It clogs arteries, puts strain on your heart, your liver and circulatory system.

If you are reading this book, you or someone you care about is probably overweight. Some may be very overweight while others may be only slightly overweight. Some of you may have ballooned in weight in the last 1-5 years, for no obvious reason. This can lead to chronic depression and a loss of self esteem. **Don't Despair! Help is at hand!** Sandra Cabot MD and nutritionist, Susie Clift B.Sc. Dip. ION., are here to help you reach a normal weight range, with compassionate and scientific advice.

Imagine getting a prescription from your doctor for a glass of grapefruit juice and watermelon whip? Scientific research shows specific foods which contain naturally occurring chemicals, can promote metabolism and aid weight reduction.

Our Philosophy

Dr Sandra Cabot and Susie Clift are **dedicated** to designing, and continually updating an effective, healthy program for your weight loss. The program supports your efforts with **compassion**, by providing "talk-back" on the **internet**. Please allow us to help you, to achieve your weight goal.

Give Yourself Mental Space

If it took 1-5 years or longer, to accumulate the excess weight that you now want to shed, it will also take some time to dispose of it. Would you like to be a size or two smaller within the next year? Perhaps within 12 months you can achieve your goal, but isn't there too much pressure on you already? Give yourself mental space to achieve your goals. Don't be too hard on yourself if you fall by the wayside-just remember that we are all human and identify those factors that may have contributed to your lapse and take measures to avoid those situations in future. Don't give up if you can't do that brisk walk around the block today, just resolve to do it tomorrow. Every effort counts, even if it is taking the stairs instead of riding on the elevator, parking half a block further from the office and walking. It all counts.

Allow yourself the mental space to discover that this eating plan is not just another diet, but a way of life to achieve your optimum weight and health. Think a little longer and examine your past pattern of weight control? Have you repeatedly tried diet after diet and only succeeded in gaining still more weight? Have you become a "yoyo" dieter and has this approach ever really worked?

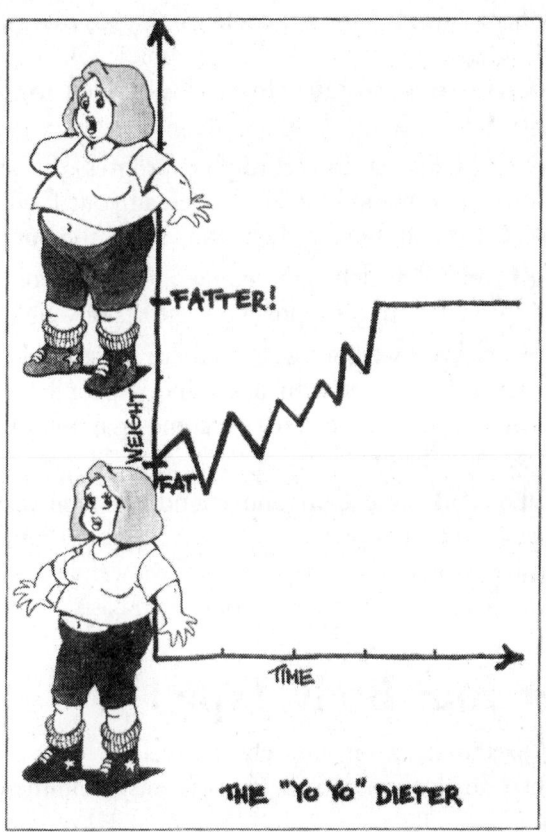

If your answer, like that of so many others is no, then isn't it time to employ a different approach? Hoping for a different result, while still employing the same attitudes, will not lead you to your goal. A new scientific, enjoyable and livable approach must be used to obtain a different result.

www.weightcontroldoctor.com

Net Weight Loss through Net Support

Net support is provided to encourage you to continue on your weight control program. When you have a problem or are just feeling low or perhaps just need a new idea on what to do next, get on the net and ask Susie Clift or have a "chin wag" in our **"on line chat room"**.

Encouragement --- we all need it!

Our **"net talk back"** will help you to focus on the positive aspects of your weight control program.

Net support for net weight loss is provided by nutritionist Susie Clift B.Sc.

A Food Diary will help you to record your progress. Susie encourages you to make note of your food intake, and email your food diary to her for helpful comments and hints to help you "stick" to your program.

"Fat Fighting Friends" which is the name of our chat room is a buddy system that has been set up to support your efforts of weight loss.

If along the route to your weight loss goal, there is a stumble, ask yourself does it really matter? Contact with like-minded people via the 'buddy system' may provide moral support to overcome disappointing behaviour, and will increase self esteem.

Dr Sandra Cabot and Susie Clift understand that your experience on weight loss programs has not been easy and a quick result has never happened; if it has, it may not have lasted. For a weight loss program to succeed, it must be easy to follow on a long term basis.

Discover your Body Type !

– Do our Questionnaire on the website called
www.weightcontroldoctor.com & get your answer immediately!

or

– Mail your photo (in swim suit or body suit) to Dr. Sandra Cabot and Mandi Timothy at SCB Inc. P.O. Box 5070 Glendale AZ 85312 – 5070

RECIPES

SOUPS

MINESTRONE SOUP

1 onion, chopped
2 potatoes, finely chopped
3 garlic cloves
15 ounces canned peeled tomatoes, finely chopped or fresh equivalent
1 tablespoon chopped parsley
2 medium carrots, chopped
1 stick celery, finely chopped
1½ cups Beef Stock
2 cups water
11 ounces canned cannellini beans

Place all ingredients except beans in a saucepan and bring to the boil. Reduce heat and simmer for 30–45 minutes; add beans and cook another 15 minutes.

Serves 6–8 (75 cal/315 kJ per serve).

ZUCCHINI SOUP

1½ pounds zucchini, sliced
2 sticks celery, finely chopped
1 carrot, finely chopped
1 potato, finely chopped
1 onion, finely chopped
2 cups water
1 cup chicken stock
½ cup soy milk
1 tablespoon chopped fresh parsley
1 tablespoon chopped fresh basil
freshly ground black pepper

Bring all ingredients except pepper, soy milk, parsley and basil to the boil in a large saucepan. Reduce heat and simmer until vegetables are just cooked. Remove from heat and blend, in blender, with soy milk. Add parsley, basil and lots of black pepper. If reheating do not boil.

Serves 6 (75 cal/315 kJ per serve).

PUMPKIN SOUP/SQUASH SOUP

1 butternut pumpkin (squash), peeled and cut into pieces
1 onion, chopped
1 potato, chopped
1 stick celery, chopped
3 garlic cloves, chopped
½ teaspoon nutmeg
1 tablespoon chopped fresh coriander, or 1 teaspoon dried
1½ cups water
1 cup Chicken Stock
½ cup soy milk
low-fat natural yoghurt and fresh parsley to garnish

Bring all ingredients except soy milk to the boil, then reduce heat and simmer until vegetables are cooked. Blend well, in blender, with soy milk and serve with a dollop of yoghurt and fresh parsley.

Serves 6–8 (150 cal/630 kJ per serve).

ITALIAN NOODLE SOUP

6½ cups water
2 small onions
1 handful Italian parsley
coriander sprigs
1 handful fresh basil
2 large potatoes
2 carrots
2 sticks celery
1 parsnip
1 turnip
1 bay leaf
small handful chives
freshly ground black pepper
½ cup presoaked red lentils
½ cup presoaked brown lentils
11 ounce can cannellini beans
26 ounce can V8 Vegetable Juice
1 garlic clove
1 tablespoon tomato paste
1 pound canned tomatoes, or fresh equivalent
1 tablespoon Vegetable Stock, mixed to a paste with some hot water
1 tablespoon low-sodium soy sauce
1⅔ cups Chicken Stock
½ cup soup noodles (small pasta)

Prepare a stock with the water, 1 onion and all vegetable skins and tops. Boil for about half an hour and strain, reserving liquid.

Blend onion, parsley, coriander and basil into a paste then combine with stock in a large pot.

Chop remaining vegetables and herbs very finely and add to stock. Add pepper, lentils, beans, V8 juice, garlic, tomato paste, tomatoes, Vegetable Stock, soy sauce and stock. Cover and cook over low heat for 1 hour. Stir pot occasionally. Add noodles and cook for an additional half hour.

Serves 8 (150 cal/630 kJ per serve).

DRESSINGS

The general rule when preparing a dressing is to start with the vinegar or juice and add the seasoning. Whisk together and slowly add the oil, a little at a time, beating as you go. Nuts and herbs should be added last.

Alternatively, you may blend oil, vinegar or juice with seasonings and then add in extras such as nuts or herbs.

A dash of water added to your salad dressing will make it go further and reduce the pungency of the vinegar.

I have significantly reduced the amount of oil that is usually requested in recipes for salad dressing, to reduce calories.

I encourage you to be creative and experiment with different types of vinegars, juices, herbs, seasonings and nuts to alter the flavour and sharpness of your dressing.

Fruit vinegars are delicious on salads that contain fruit.

You may simply wish to squeeze a little fresh lemon or lime juice over your salad. This will increase your vitamin C levels and add a few extra enzymes to aid digestion.

SPICY THAI DRESSING

2 stalks lemon grass, chopped
3 chillies, seeded if desired, chopped
1/4 cup lime or lemon juice
1 tablespoon fish sauce

30 cal/130 kJ/1/3 cup

GINGER DRESSING

1/3 cup lime juice
1 tablespoon fish sauce
1 teaspoon brown sugar
1 teaspoon ground ginger

40 cal/168 kJ/1/3 cup

SWEET LIME DRESSING

1 tablespoon fish sauce
1 dessertspoon sugar
2 tablespoons lime juice

70 cal/294 kJ/1/3 cup

TANGY LIME DRESSING

2 tablespoons lime juice
1 tablespoons lime zest
2 tablespoons fish sauce

40 cal/168 kJ/1/3 cup

MUSTARD VINAIGRETTE

2 teaspoons light oil
juice of 1 lime or lemon
1 teaspoon French mustard
1 garlic clove, finely chopped

120 cal/504 kJ/1/2 cup

NO OIL DRESSING

½ cup red wine vinegar
juice of 1 lemon or lime
2 garlic cloves, finely chopped
chives, chopped
freshly ground black pepper

40 cal/168 kJ

MOCK SOUR CREAM DRESSING

½ cup skimmed ricotta cheese
¼ cup plain low-fat yoghurt
chives, chopped
parsley and mint if desired

240 cal/1008 kJ

CORIANDER MAYONNAISE

½ cup low-fat yoghurt
⅓ cup light mayonnaise
coriander, chopped
2 teaspoons French mustard
2 teaspoons lemon juice
freshly ground black pepper

300 cal/1260 kJ

SWEET WALNUT DRESSING

1 tablespoon light olive oil
1 tablespoon lemon, lime, grapefruit
  or orange juice
2 tablespoons coarsely chopped walnuts
½ teaspoon honey
2 garlic cloves, finely chopped

300 cal/1260 kJ

VINAIGRETTE DRESSING

1 tablespoon light olive oil
1 tablespoon white wine vinegar or
  lemon juice
1 garlic clove, finely chopped
freshly ground black pepper

200 cal/840 kJ

HAZELNUT DRESSING

1 tablespoon light olive oil
1 tablespoon balsamic vinegar
2 teaspoons water
2 tablespoons coarsely chopped
  roasted hazelnuts
½ teaspoon ground ginger
½ teaspoon honey

300 cal/1260 kJ

RASPBERRY VINAIGRETTE

2 teaspoons raspberry vinegar
1 teaspoon lime juice
½ teaspoon dijon mustard
1 tablespoon olive oil
2 tablespoons coarsely chopped
  pecan nuts

300 cal/1260 kJ

SAUCES

EASY ONION SAUCE

3 cups chopped onion
1 tablespoon skim milk or soy milk
½ teaspoon nutmeg

freshly ground black pepper to taste
1 desertspoon lemon juice

Microwave or steam the onion and blend with the milk, nutmeg, black pepper and a dash of lemon juice.

•*Great to serve with chicken, fish or vegetables.*

Serves 4 (35 cal/147 kJ per serve).

CHILLI SAUCE

1 chopped tomato
1 spring onion, finely chopped
1 seeded and chopped fresh chilli or
  ½ teaspoon dried chilli

1 dessertspoon finely chopped
  parsley
1 dessertspoon finely chopped
  coriander

Combine all ingredients and cook until tender in microwave, or in saucepan stirring constantly over moderate heat.

Serves 1 (35 cal/147 kJ).

BLENDER HOLLANDAISE

1 tablespoon olive oil

1 egg yolk
juice of 1 or 2 limes or lemons

Blend all ingredients. Use immediately, it will not keep.

Serves 3 (approximately 50 cal/210 kJ per serve).

PARSLEY SAUCE

1 dessertspoon olive oil
1 tablespoon wholemeal flour
1¼ cups low-fat calcium enriched milk
1 tablespoon finely chopped parsley

freshly ground black pepper
a squeeze of lemon juice and 1 teaspoon of grated lemon rind
onion or shallots, finely chopped (optional)

Warm oil in a small saucepan. Add flour away from heat and stir with a wooden spoon until smooth. Stir over low heat for 1 minute, it must not burn. Add milk gradually, stirring well until sauce boils and thickens. Add parsley, lemon juice, lemon rind and finely chopped onion or shallots if desired.

Serves 6 (approximately 50 cal/210 kJ per serve).

PESTO SAUCE

½ bunch fresh basil
1 tablespoon pine nuts
2 garlic cloves

2 teaspoons olive oil
freshly ground black pepper

Blend all ingredients and serve on cooked pasta or jacket potatoes.

Serves 2 (approximately 75 cal/315 kJ per serve).

BASIC FOUNDATION SAUCE

2 tablespoon olive oil
2 tablespoons flour
1½ cups low-fat calcium enriched

milk or soy milk (or a combination for a creamier low-fat sauce that does not have a strong soy taste)

Warm oil over low heat and stir in flour. Cook for 2 minutes over low heat, stirring continuously. Add milk gradually and stir until the sauce boils and thickens.

•This basic recipe is useful as a base for any sauce. Add less milk to make a thicker binding sauce for pies or fritters.

Serves 4 (approximately 110 cal/462 kJ per serve). Total calories for sauce are approximately 440/1848 kJ.

VARIATIONS FOR BASIC FOUNDATION SAUCE

Many herbs can be added to change the sauce according to the food it is to accompany. Listed below are a few simple sauce ideas.

Mustard Sauce—Add 3 teaspoons of prepared mustard to sauce, serve with beef or fish. Total: 460 cal/1932 kJ.

Egg Sauce—Add 2 chopped hard boiled eggs to sauce. Serve with fish, chicken or beef. Total: 680 cal/2856 kJ.

Mushroom Sauce—Cook ½ cup of mushrooms and a little garlic in the microwave and add to sauce. Total: 460 cal/1932 kJ.

Florentine Sauce—Add a dash of tabasco, Worcestershire sauce, nutmeg, parsley and 1 cup of cooked, pureed spinach. Serve with fish, eggs, chicken or potato. Total: 490 cal/2058 kJ.

Mornay Sauce—Add 2 tablespoons low-fat cheese and a sprinkle of Parmesan to the sauce as it thickens. Serve with fish, seafood, eggs and vegetables. Total: 670 cal/2814 kJ.

Onion Sauce—Steam or microwave 2 finely chopped onions until tender, and stir into sauce. Good with beef or fish. Total: 500 cal/2100 kJ.

TOMATO SALSA

2 tomatoes, finely chopped
¼ capsicum, finely chopped
1 small onion, finely chopped
3 or 4 fresh basil leaves, finely
   chopped

fresh parsley, chopped
½ fresh chilli with seeds removed,
   finely chopped

Combine all ingredients in a small bowl.

Serves 2 (approximately 45 cal/189 kJ per serve).

MINTED TOMATO SALSA

2 tomatoes, finely chopped
1 small onion, finely chopped
1 dessertspoon fresh mint, finely
   chopped

1 dessertspoon fresh parsley, finely
   chopped

Combine all ingredients in a small bowl.

Serves 2 (approximately 35 cal/147 kJ per serve).

APPETIZERS

STUFFED MUSHROOM CAPS

Allow 3 mushrooms for each person.

Remove stems and wipe caps with a damp cloth. Place upside-down in a shallow baking dish ready for filling.

SAUCE
1 tablespoon warmed olive oil
1 tablespoon wholemeal flour
1 cup low-fat milk or soy milk

½ bunch freshly cooked asparagus or 12 ounce can asparagus pieces, drained
paprika

Combine oil and flour in a small saucepan and stir over moderate heat for 1 minute. Add milk and continue stirring until mixture boils and thickens. Add cooked asparagus pieces and blend. Fill or cover mushrooms and sprinkle with paprika. Bake or grill until hot and bubbly.

85 cal/357 kJ per serve

EGG AND TUNA COMBO

2 hard-boiled eggs, chopped
8 ounces tuna in spring water, drained and mashed with a fork
½ cup low fat cottage cheese
1 shallot, finely chopped

1 dessertspoon chopped fresh dill
1 dessertspoon chopped fresh parsley
cayenne pepper or paprika (optional)

Combine all ingredients and serve with toasted wholemeal bread, crackers or pita bread.

Total calories excluding bread approximately 475/1995 kJ.

DEVILLED EGGS

6 free range eggs
1 dessertspoon light mayonnaise
1 teaspoon dijon mustard

1 teaspoon curry powder
fresh mint and parsley, finely
  chopped, to garnish

Hard-boil the eggs, shell them and allow to cool. Cut eggs in half, lengthwise, and remove yolks. Mash the yolks with the other ingredients in a small bowl and place spoonfuls back into each egg half. Garnish with a little parsley and mint.

Serves 6 (approximately 80 cal/336 kJ per serve).

GUACAMOLE

1 medium avocado
3 garlic cloves, finely chopped
lemon or lime juice to taste

Mash avocado and garlic together with a fork. Mix in some lemon or lime juice to flavour the dish. Guacamole mixture should have a smooth but firm consistency. You may add a little fresh chilli to this recipe if desired.

Serves 2–4 (total calories approximately 500/2100 kJ).

This recipe can be used as a dip with unsalted crackers or fresh chopped raw vegetables. I suggest a platter that contains broccoli florets, carrot sticks, zucchini sticks, capsicum, celery, fennel and radish. A large plateful of these vegetables would yield about 80 to 100 calories.

HUMMUS (HOUMMOS)

10 to 11 ounces cooked chick peas
⅓ cup tahini (sesame paste)
3 garlic cloves, chopped

juice of 2–3 lemons
freshly ground black pepper

Blend or grind chickpeas until smooth. Add all other ingredients to blender, and combine thoroughly.

Add more tahini or lemon juice as necessary, to suit your taste and to reach a smooth, but not runny consistency. Place into a serving dish and sprinkle with paprika if desired.

This vegetarian dish is an excellent addition to a salad, can be eaten as a dip or an alternative spread on crackers or bread. It is a good source of protein, calcium and vitamin C.

1 tablespoon contains 60 cal/252 kJ.

BABAGANOUJ

2 pounds eggplant
3 garlic cloves
juice of 2 lemons

⅓ cup tahini (sesame paste)
roasted sesame seeds to garnish

Bake in a moderate oven 350°F or grill whole eggplants (if grilling use small eggplants) until the skin blisters and turns black (30 minutes). Peel eggplants while they are still hot.

Blend the eggplant pulp with the garlic, lemon juice and tahini. You may wish to taste the mixture and add more lemon juice or garlic to suit your palate. Place in a dish, sprinkle with roasted sesame seeds and chill.

Serve with pita bread, rice crackers or fresh raw vegetables.

Serves 6–8 (approximately 70 cal/294 kJ per serve).

SALADS

TABBOULI SALAD

1 cup bulgur or cracked wheat
3 shallots, chopped
1 bunch parsley, about 4 ounces, finely chopped

½ cup finely chopped fresh mint
juice of 2 lemons
3 tomatoes, finely chopped

Place bulgur in a bowl and cover with cold water. Leave to soak for 30 minutes. Drain, press out excess water and leave to dry for 30 minutes.

Place bulgur in a bowl and combine with the other ingredients. Lightly toss, and serve immediately.

Serves 4 (approximately 75 cal/315 kJ per serve).

FRESH ASPARAGUS VINAIGRETTE

12 fresh asparagus spears

DRESSING
1 tablespoon pine nuts
2 shallots, finely chopped
1 dessertspoon finely chopped fresh tarragon or parsley

1 garlic clove, finely chopped
1 tablespoon olive oil
1 tablespoon white wine vinegar or lime juice
1 teaspoon honey

Trim thick, coarse end, from asparagus. Lightly steam, taking care not to overcook. Rinse quickly under cold water to retain colour and arrange on serving platter.

Lightly roast pine nuts in microwave or skillet and set aside. Combine all other ingredients in a glass container and whisk lightly. Pour over the asparagus and scatter pine nuts on top.

Serves 4 (approximately 75 cal/315 kJ per serve).

GREEN VEGETABLE PLATE

Arrange a combination of raw and steamed green vegetables on a platter or large dinner plate. A good combination would be:

4 spears fresh asparagus	4 button squash
8 snow peas	½ sliced avocado
8 whole green beans	raw zucchini sticks
4 broccoli florets	

Serves 4–6 (approximately 70 cal/294 kJ per serve).

DUKKAH

In a heavy skillet, roast a combination of coarsely chopped pine nuts, cashews, hazelnuts or macadamia nuts, sesame and sunflower seeds. Add 1 teaspoon of lightly crushed, roasted coriander seeds and mix together. Combined quantity ½ cup. Place in a small bowl and serve with vegetables.

Serves 4 (approximately 125 cal/525 kJ per serve).

•*Our Mustard Vinaigrette (see page 00) may be served with this dish.*

MIXED BEAN AND RICE SALAD

½ cup canned four bean mix	1 handful fresh parsley, finely chopped
1 cup cooked brown rice, cold	
1 medium onion, finely chopped	A few sundried tomatoes, finely sliced
3 shallots, finely chopped	
½ red pepper, thinly sliced	¼ cup raisins
½ cup corn kernels	¼ cup Hazelnut Dressing (recipe page 148)

Combine all salad ingredients in a serving bowl, add dressing and toss well.

Serves 2 (approximately 400 cal/1680 kJ per serve).

PASTA SALAD

2 cups cooked macaroni
1 stick celery, finely chopped
8 cherry tomatoes, halved
2 tablespoons chopped parsley
2 shallots, finely chopped

½ red pepper, thinly sliced
3 radish, sliced
⅓ cup sliced mushroom
2 small sliced zucchini
5 tablespoons Vinaigrette Dressing (recipe page 148)

Combine all ingredients in a serving bowl, add dressing and toss well.

Serves 4 (approximately 170 cal/714 kJ per serve).

BEET AND WATERCRESS SALAD

1 bunch watercress or arugula
2 medium beets
2 large red onions

6 radishes
lettuce leaves

Cook and slice fresh beets, leave to cool. Thinly slice onions and place in a bowl. Pour over some boiling water and let stand for 1 minute, then drain.

Arrange lettuce leaves in a bowl or on a plate. Top with beets, onion, watercress and sliced radish. Sprinkle with dressing of your choice or fresh lemon juice.

Serves 8 (approximately 20 cal/84 kJ per serve).

GREEN BEAN AND APPLE SALAD

1 large grannysmith apple
¼ cup No Oil Dressing (recipe page 148)
One pound green beans, topped and tailed
1 red onion, thinly sliced
1 red pepper, sliced or chopped

1 tablespoon finely chopped fresh parsley
1 tablespoon finely chopped fresh mint
6 lettuce leaves
1 cup snow pea sprouts or alfalfa sprouts

Core apple, dice into bite-sized cubes and place in a small bowl. Pour over No Oil Dressing, leave to sit while you wash and prepare other ingredients.

Place all ingredients in a large bowl and toss lightly.

Serves 8 (approximately 60 cal/252 kJ per serve).

CARROT AND RAISIN SALAD

3 large carrots, grated
¼ green pepper, chopped
⅓ cup seedless raisins

1 tablespoon sunflower seeds.
2 tablespoons Sweet Walnut
 Dressing, made with orange
 juice (recipe page 148)

Combine all ingredients and toss well with dressing.

Serves 6 (approximately 60 cal/252 kJ per serve).

SPINACH AND WALNUT SALAD

6 spinach leaves, stems removed
nutmeg (optional)
3 shallots, finely chopped
¼ cup Sweet Walnut Dressing
 (recipe page 148)

Lightly steam spinach for 2 minutes, chop coarsely and set aside to cool. Sprinkle with a little nutmeg if desired. Lightly toss shallots and dressing through spinach.

Serves 6 (approximately 60 cal/252 kJ per serve).

•*Some raisins or sultanas are a nice addition to this salad.*

SLIMMERS' EGG AND POTATO SALAD

3 large potatoes, brushed, diced
 and cooked
1 onion, finely chopped
4 boiled eggs, sliced
1 tablespoon finely chopped parsley

1 tablespoon finely chopped mint
1 cup plain natural low-fat yoghurt
sprinkle cayenne pepper
green pepper rings to garnish

Combine all ingredients in a large bowl and lightly toss. Garnish with green pepper rings.

Serves 6 (approximately 125 cal/525 kJ per serve).

GREEK SALAD

2 cups shredded lettuce
1 tomato, thinly sliced
1 small cucumber, sliced
½ red pepper, sliced
1 onion, thinly sliced
4 ounces fetta cheese, cut into
small cubes

8 black olives
½ cup No Oil Dressing (recipe page 148)
fresh mint, finely chopped to garnish
fresh parsley, finely chopped to garnish
fresh basil, finely chopped to garnish

Arrange a bed of lettuce on a large plate. Place a layer of sliced tomatoes on top, followed by sliced cucumber, capsicum and onion. Top with fetta cheese and olives. Pour dressing over and sprinkle with fresh herbs.

Serves 2 (approximately 265 cal/1113 kJ per serve).

MUSHROOM AND SNOW PEA SALAD

4 ½ ounces mushrooms
12 snow peas
2 spring onions, sliced
juice of 1 lemon or lime

2 teaspoons oil
8 roasted hazelnuts, roughly chopped

Wipe mushrooms, trim stems and slice thinly. Place in a bowl with washed, whole snow peas and spring onion. Combine lemon juice and oil and pour over salad vegetables. Sprinkle over hazelnuts and lightly toss salad.

Serves 2 (approximately 100 cal/420 kJ per serve).

CALAMARI AND SEA SCALLOPS THAI SALAD

1 pound calamari
½ pound sea scallops
Marinade
½ cup lime juice
1 tablespoon fish sauce or soy sauce

2 stalks of lemon grass, finely chopped
3 shallots, finely chopped
2 red chillies, seeded and sliced

Clean calamari and thinly slice into rings. Wash scallops. Bring a saucepan of water to the boil and quickly cook calamari rings and scallops. Drain and set aside.

Combine all marinade ingredients in a large bowl and add cooked calamari and scallops. Marinate for 15 minutes and then serve on a bed of hot rice.

Serves 4 (120 cal/504 kJ per serve; 300 cal/1260 kJ per serve with ¾ cup rice).

•Boiled calamari is not tough or chewy and is simple to prepare. The combination of it with the marinade makes a delicious meal that leaves your taste buds tingling.

SEAFOOD SALAD

4 ounces cooked fish or shellfish/canned or fresh, roughly chopped
2 shallots, finely chopped
½ inch ginger root, finely chopped
1 red chilli, seeded and finely chopped

8 roasted cashew nuts, roughly chopped
1 mango roughly chopped
¼ cup Tangy Lime Dressing (recipe page 147)
Lettuce leaves
Cherry tomatoes and mint leaves to garnish

Combine all ingredients together in a medium bowl with dressing. Serve immediately on washed lettuce leaves. Garnish with cherry tomatoes and mint leaves. Serve with rice if desired.
Serves 2 (225 cal/945 kJ per serve; 405 cal/1701 kJ per serve with ¾ cup rice).
*Sardines can be substituted for the fish/shellfish.

LIME CHICKEN SALAD

2 chicken breasts, grilled and cut into small cubes
2 shallots, finely chopped
½ green pepper, finely chopped
2 red chillies, seeded and finely chopped

lettuce leaves
1 tablespoon chopped mint
¼ cup Sweet Lime Dressing (recipe page 147)
freshly ground black pepper

Combine chicken, shallots, green pepper and chillies in a medium bowl. Toss with dressing, then serve on washed lettuce leaves and garnish with mint. Sprinkle with pepper. Serve with rice if desired.

Serves 4 (155 cal/651 kJ per serve; 335 cal/407 kJ per serve with ¾ cup rice).

PAPAYA AND CHICKEN SALAD

2 chicken breasts, grilled and cut into small cubes
2 tablespoons roughly chopped almonds
1 small or ½ large pawpaw, cut into cubes or small balls
2 red chillies, seeded and finely chopped
3 shallots, chopped
1 tablespoon chopped fresh mint or coriander
½ cup Ginger Dressing (recipe page 147)

Combine all ingredients in a bowl and lightly toss with dressing. Serve with steamed or boiled rice.

Serves 4 (190 cal/798 kJ per serve; 370 cal/1554 kJ per serve with ¾ cup rice).

CUCUMBER SALAD

2 medium cucumbers
1 dessertspoon sugar
2 tablespoons white vinegar
1 red chilli, seed and finely chopped
1 heaped tablespoon roughly chopped almonds or pecan nuts
2 shallots, finely chopped
1 tablespoon chopped fresh coriander

Wash cucumbers and slice horizontally through the middle. Leave the skin on and carefully scoop out the seeds. Finely slice the cucumber and place in a serving bowl.

Combine sugar and vinegar and stir until sugar has dissolved. Pour over cucumber and mix well.

Sprinkle chilli, nuts, shallots and coriander on top, and leave to marinate for 1 hour.

Serves 4 (approximately 60 cal/252 kJ per serve).

•*Cucumbers are rich in vitamin A, potassium, calcium and phosphorus. This dish from Thailand turns a simple vegetable into a very tasty, refreshing salad.*

ENTRÉES

TANDOORI FISH

1 medium onion
6 garlic cloves
¾ inch fresh ginger root
1 chilli
juice of 1 lemon
1 tablespoon ground coriander
1 teaspoon cumin
2 teaspoons fennel seeds

5 cardamon pods
1 teaspoon ground cinnamon
freshly ground black pepper
1 teaspoon paprika
1 cup low-fat natural yoghurt
1 whole fish, about 2-2.5 pounds
lime slices to garnish
fresh coriander to garnish

Blend onion, garlic, ginger and chilli with a powerful blender until smooth.

Combine all other spices and herbs in a mortar and pestle and grind together. Add spices and yoghurt to onion mixture and blend to a paste.

Make several diagonal incisions across the fish and rub on paste, inside and out, to coat fish. Refrigerate for 2 hours.

Grill, barbecue or bake the fish until the skin is crisp and the flesh begins to flake—about 20 minutes depending on size of fish.

Garnish with slices of lime and fresh coriander.

Serves 2–4 (approximately 400 cal/1680 kJ per serve).
* Commercial tandoori mixture is available in some supermarkets and health food stores.

CREAMY FISH ROLLS WITH DILL SAUCE

8 thin white fish fillets
1 tablespoon finely chopped
 parsley and ½ inch piece finely
 chopped fresh ginger mixed into
 the juice of 1 lime or lemon

8 slices of fresh mango or 8 large
 pawpaw pieces
1 cup low-fat calcium-enriched milk
2 teaspoons cornflour
1 tablespoon chopped fresh dill

Brush 1 side of each fish fillet with lime juice mixture. Roll each fillet (brushed side to middle) around a slice of fruit and secure with a tooth-pick or skewer. Place in a single layer in a shallow ovenproof dish. Pour over milk, cover and poach in microwave for about 8 minutes, or in moderate oven, 425° F, for 15–20 minutes until fish is just cooked. DO NOT OVERCOOK. Carefully remove fish rolls with a slotted spoon and set aside in a warm place while sauce is made from pan juices.

Blend cornflour with a little cold low-fat calcium-enriched milk to make a smooth paste. Strain pan juices and place in a small saucepan. Add blended cornflour and stir constantly over moderate heat until mixture boils and thickens. Add fresh chopped dill and serve immediately over fish rolls.

•*The enzymes in the fruit and fresh ginger in this recipe assist your digestion. If you dislike combining fruit with fish then try using carrot and zucchini straws or oysters as a filling instead.*

Serves 8 (approximately 200 cal/840 kJ per serve).

BAKED WHOLE FISH WITH FRUIT FILLING

1 cup cooked brown rice
2 shallots, chopped
⅓ cup chopped celery
fresh chilli (optional)
½ inch piece fresh ginger
fresh pieces of pawpaw or mango or rockmelon (many fruits may be used in this recipe, the choice is yours)

2 to 3 pounds whole fish such as snapper, rainbow trout or perch
lemon or lime juice
fennel tips, slices of lemon or lime and some fresh ginger cut into thin slices to garnish

In a small bowl combine cooked rice, shallots, celery, chilli, ginger and fresh fruit. Stuff cleaned and scaled fish with this mixture and place in a baking dish. Squeeze over fresh lemon or lime juice and garnish with fennel, ginger and citrus slices. Pour ¼ cup water into dish and cover with foil or lid to stop fish drying out. Bake in a moderate oven 350° F until fish is just cooked approximately 35 minutes.

Serves 4 (approximately 200 cal/840 kJ per serve).

PORK AND PINEAPPLE KEBABS

3 ounces lean pork fillet
2 slices fresh pineapple
1 onion

4 fresh mushrooms
6 cherry tomatoes

Cut all ingredients except tomatoes into bite-sized pieces and thread alternately onto bamboo or metal skewers. Grill or barbecue until meat is cooked to your liking.

Serves 1 (approximately 240 cal/1008 kJ).

LAMB AND FRUIT KEBABS

3.5 ounces lamb steak
3 apricots or 1 small mango
1 onion

4 fresh mushrooms
6 cherry tomatoes

Cut all ingredients except tomatoes into bite-sized pieces and thread alternately onto bamboo or metal skewers. Grill or barbecue until meat is cooked to your liking.

Serves 1 (approximately 230 cal/966 kJ).

SATAY CHICKEN KEBABS

1 onion
2 red chillies
1 tablespoon fish sauce
2 teaspoons cumin
1 teaspoon turmeric

2 teaspoons ginger powder
2 teaspoons black peppercorns
1 teaspoon brown sugar
2 garlic cloves
6 inches lemon grass, finely chopped
3 chicken breasts

Blend onion, chillies and fish sauce until smooth. Combine all other ingredients except chicken in a mortar and pestle and pound together well, breaking up the peppercorns and lemon grass. Add this mixture into the onion mixture and blend again. This is your marinade.

Trim all fat from chicken and cut into bite-sized pieces. Place meat in marinade and make sure you coat each piece of chicken well. Marinate for 1 hour.

Thread chicken onto bamboo skewers and grill or barbecue until cooked.

Serves 6 (145 cal/609 kJ per serve).

BRAISED STEAK

12 ounces skirt steak or stew beef
3 sticks celery
2 large carrots
2 medium onions

mixed herbs
1½ cups Beef Stock
½ cup water

Cut steak into 8 serves and slice vegetables into large pieces. Heat a little water in a large casserole dish over moderate heat. Quickly brown the meat in the water to seal in the juices and set aside.

Place vegetables, herbs, stock and the water into the casserole dish. Stir to combine and place meat carefully on top, in order to cook it above the vegetables. Seal with a tight fitting lid and bring to the boil.

Reduce heat and simmer with the lid on for 2 hours.

Serves 4 (approximately 200 cal/840 kJ per serve).

IRISH STEW

12 small potatoes
3 carrots
1 teaspoon Vegetable Stock
½ cup warm water
4 sprigs fresh oregano
1 bunch finely chopped parsley

3 onions
2½ pounds lamb steaks or fillets
4 tomatoes or 1 can tomatoes
1 tablespoon low-sodium soy sauce
freshly ground black pepper
2 sticks celery, finely chopped

Scrub potatoes and carrots. Cut potatoes in half and line the bottom of a large casserole dish or saucepan with them. Disolve the stock in the warm water and pour over. Sprinkle with a handful of herbs and arrange a layer of the finely sliced onion rings. Place meat on top, then the tomatoes, followed by soy sauce, pepper and remaining vegetables and herbs. Cover with a tight fitting lid and cook over low heat for 1½–2 hours (on a heat pad if possible). Give the pot a light shake every 15 minutes to prevent burning.

Serves 8 (approximately 375 cal/1575 kJ per serve).

CHICKEN AND VEGETABLE HOTPOT

3¾ cups tomato or V8 vegetable juice

12 potatoes, scrubbed and halved

½ bunch fresh basil, finely chopped

1 handful fresh parsley, finely chopped

freshly ground black pepper

2 sticks celery, chopped

2 large onions, sliced

8 chicken thigh fillets, trimmed of fat

32 ounces canned tomatoes or fresh equivalent, chopped

3 carrots, chopped

2 zucchinis, chopped

1 parsnip, chopped

12 ounces pumpkin, chopped

2 bay leaves

2 tablespoons low-sodium soy sauce

1 large teaspoon Vegetable Stock powder dissolved in a ½ cup of water

½ pound green beans, topped and tailed

Pour a little V8 Vegetable Juice into the bottom of a heavy based saucepan. Arrange the potatoes over the bottom of the pot and sprinkle with some of the basil, parsley and black pepper. Next, arrange some celery and onion rings over the herbs, followed by the chicken fillets. Pour over half the chopped tomatoes. Arrange carrots, zucchinis, parsnip and pumpkin in layers, with the onions on top of this, sprinkling with remaining basil, parsley and black pepper as you go. Pour over remaining tomatoes and add bay leaves, soy sauce and dissolved vegetable stock. Lastly place green beans on top. Check the level of juice in the pot, it should be one inch below the highest layer of the vegetables (add more V8 Vegetable Juice if needed).

Cover and cook over low heat, on heat pad if you have one, for 1½–2 hours. At 15-minute intervals you must come and shake the pot, lid on and all. It is an old Italian custom!

Serves 8 (approximately 350 cal/1470 kJ per serve).

CHICKEN AND MUSHROOM PIE

PIE CRUST
1½ cups cooked brown rice
1 dessertspoon oil
1 tablespoon chopped parsley
1 tablespoon sesame seeds

SAUCE
1 dessertspoon olive oil
1 tablespoon flour
freshly ground black pepper
1 clove garlic, chopped
¼ cup low-fat calcium-enriched milk or soy milk
¼ cup chicken stock

FILLING
1 pound cooked chicken, cut into bite-sized pieces, with skin, bones and any visible fat removed.

2 tablespoons thinly sliced red capsicum
½ cup chopped broccoli florets
4 shallots, finely chopped
4 ounces fresh mushrooms
2 tablespoons chopped fresh parsley
1 dessertspoon chopped fresh rosemary or basil (1 teaspoon dry)
(if you have any left over cooked vegetables they may be added to this dish)

TOPPING
1 cup cooked, mashed sweet potato and sesame seeds

To prepare sauce, warm oil over low heat. Add flour, pepper and garlic away from heat and stir until combined well with oil. Return to heat and stir over low heat for 1 minute. Add milk and stock and stir continuously until sauce boils and thickens.

In a large bowl combine all the filling ingredients (plus extra vegetables if desired) and stir in the prepared sauce. Fill pie crust with mixture, top with mashed sweet potato and sprinkle with sesame seeds. Bake in a moderate oven 350° F for 30–40 minutes.

Serves 6 (225 cal/945 kJ per serve).

AVOCADO AND CHICKEN IN FILO

2 chicken breasts, cut in half
8 sheets filo pastry
⅓ cup low-fat natural yoghurt
1 small avocado, sliced
lemon juice
freshly ground black pepper

tarragon, basil or marjoram
2 tablespoons oil
1 tablespoon sesame seeds

Lightly pound chicken breasts to an even thickness. Brush one sheet of filo with a little yoghurt and cover with a second sheet. Brush again and fold in half to form a square. Place a piece of chicken diagonally at corner of pastry and top with avocado slices, lemon juice, pepper and your choice of herbs. Fold in half, roll up into a pastry parcel, tucking ends under as you go. Repeat with remaining chicken and filo. Place on a lightly greased baking tray and brush with a little warm oil. Sprinkle with sesame seeds and bake in a moderate oven for 20–25 minutes or until pastry is golden brown.

Serves 4 (approximately 350 cal/1470 kJ per serve).

CABBAGE ROLLS

¼ cup buckwheat
8 cabbage leaves
1 cup cooked chickpeas
½ cup low-fat yoghurt
1 cup cooked brown rice
½ cup chopped fresh mushrooms
½ cup chopped celery
2 shallots, finely chopped
1 tablespoon chopped parsley
1 tablespoon chopped mint

1 tablespoon chopped fresh
marjoram or chopped basil
(1 teaspoon dried)

SAUCE
3 large ripe tomatoes or 1 pound canned peeled tomatoes
1 onion, finely chopped
1 tablespoon fresh majoram or fresh basil

Soak buckwheat in warm water for 30 minutes to soften. Strain and set aside. Trim thick stalks from cabbage leaves and steam until just tender. Do not overcook.

Puree chickpeas in a blender with the yoghurt. In a large bowl, combine chickpea puree, brown rice, buckwheat, mushrooms, celery, shallots and herbs. Divide mixture into 8 portions and place each portion onto a precooked cabbage leaf. Fold and roll up the mixture into each leaf, tucking in the ends as you go to form small parcels. Place in a single layer in a casserole dish.

To prepare sauce puree tomatoes in a blender and add onion and basil or marjoram. Pour sauce over the rolls, cover and bake in a moderate oven for 30 minutes.

Serves 4 (approximately 225 cal/945 kJ per serve).

KIDNEY BEAN BAKE

9 ounces canned red kidney beans, drained
1 carrot, grated
1 stick celery, finely chopped
1 cup ricotta cheese
1 tablespoon finely chopped parsley

1 dessertspoon finely chopped fresh basil
freshly ground black pepper
2 onions, finely sliced
⅔ cup vegetable stock
2 cups cooked, mashed sweet potato
roasted sesame seeds

To the drained beans mix in the grated carrot and celery. Lightly mix ricotta cheese, parsley, basil and black pepper together.

Steam the onions until soft.

Put a third of the bean mixture into a greased ovenproof dish. Top with half the sliced onions and half the ricotta cheese. Repeat with another layer of beans and remaining onion and ricotta. Finish with a layer of beans. Pour over vegetable stock. Top with mashed sweet potato and sprinkle over sesame seeds. Bake in a moderate oven for 30 minutes.

Serves 4 (approximately 260 cal/1092 kJ per serve).

OVEN-BAKED FALAFEL

¼ cup buckwheat
7 ounces cooked chick peas
1 onion, finely chopped
2 shallots, finely chopped
3 garlic cloves, chopped
1 tablespoon chopped parsley

1 dessertspoon chopped mint
fresh coriander (optional)
freshly ground black pepper
¼ cup wholemeal flour
1 egg
1 tablespoon lemon juice
¼ cup sesame seeds

Soak buckwheat in hot water for 10 minutes and drain well.

Finely grind or blend chick peas and add all other ingredients, except sesame seeds, and mix thoroughly. Cover and chill for 1 hour.

With wet hands, shape mixture into individual patties and roll them in sesame seeds. Let sit a further 10 minutes and bake in a moderate oven until golden brown.

Serves 6 (approximately 55 cal/231 kJ per serve).

•*Traditionally from the Middle East, falafels are delicious served with flat bread, houmos (recipe page 00) and tabbouli. This combination of foods provides a good source of protein and calcium.*

Falafels are usually deep fried, so take care with calories if you have not made them yourself.

SOY BEAN PATTIES

One pound canned soy beans, drained and mashed or coarsely blended with 1 tablespoon tahini (sesame paste)
½ cup pre-soaked buckwheat or cooked brown rice
1 stick celery, finely chopped
1 carrot, grated

1 onion, finely chopped
3 garlic cloves, finely chopped
1 tablespoon chopped fresh parsley
1 tablespoon chopped fresh coriander
freshly ground black pepper
1 egg
sesame seeds

Mix together all ingredients except sesame seeds. Add some wholemeal flour if mixture is too sloppy. Form into patties and roll in sesame seeds. Refrigerate for 15 minutes so patties hold together better when cooking. Cook in non-stick pan with a smear of olive oil until golden brown, turning once.

•*It is possible to substitute other beans or lentils in this recipe without affecting calories.*

Makes 10–12 patties (approximately 100 cal/420 kJ per patty).

QUICK MEXICAN BEANS

15 ounces canned red kidney beans, drained
15 ounces peeled tomatoes, roughly chopped
½ pepper, chopped
1 onion, chopped
1 carrot, grated
1 stick celery, finely chopped
¾ cup water
1 dessertspoon chopped fresh basil

Place all of the ingredients in a saucepan and cook until tender and thick (approximately 30 minutes), stirring occasionally.

Serves 6 (approximately 100 cal/420 kJ per serve).

DAHL

3 cups water
½ pound red lentils
1 potato, diced
3.5 ounces sweet potato, diced
3.5 ounces pumpkin, diced
1 onion, finely chopped
3 teaspoons curry powder or paste
1 tablespoon low-sodium soy sauce

Heat water until boiling, then add lentils, vegetables, curry and soy sauce. Reduce heat and cook until vegetables are soft and the dahl has thickened (about 20–30 minutes), stirring occasionally. Blend until smooth and serve.

•*Any vegetables can be used in this dish. Dahl is a good source of protein when combined with brown rice.*

Serves 2–4 (approximately 250 cal/1050 kJ per serve; 500 cal altogether).

BUTTERNUT AND CASHEW QUICHE

PIE CRUST

1½ cups cooked brown rice
1 tablespoon chopped parsley
1 dessertspoon oil
1 tablespoon sesame seeds

FILLING

6 eggs
½ cup low-fat soy milk

1½ cups steamed butternut pumpkin, cut into small cubes
⅓ cup raw cashews
2 shallots and/or chives, finely chopped
1½ cups your choice of chopped raw green vegetables (zucchini, broccoli, green beans, peas or capsicum)
pinch of nutmeg

Combine all pie crust ingredients and press into an ungreased pie dish.

Beat together eggs and milk. Pour into uncooked pie crust and sprinkle in other ingredients. Flavour with fresh herbs such as tarragon, dill or parsley (if using dried herbs use sparingly as they are much stronger in flavour and can overpower the subtle flavours of this dish).

Sprinkle with a little paprika and bake in a moderate oven for 30 minutes.

Serves 6 (approximately 235 cal/987 kJ per serve).

QUICK CURRIED EGGS

4 hard-boiled eggs, sliced

SAUCE

1 dessertspoon olive oil
1 tablespoon wholemeal flour

1 cup soy milk
mild curry herbs (to taste)
freshly ground black pepper
fresh parsley, chopped, to garnish

Arrange the sliced eggs in a shallow dish.

Warm oil over low heat and add flour. Stir continuously for 1 minute until combined. Add soy milk and continue stirring until mixture boils and thickens. Add curry herbs and pour mixture over eggs. Sprinkle with fresh chopped parsley.

Serves 2 (275 cal/1155 kJ per serve).

SLIMMERS' SPAGHETTI BOLOGNAISE

2 onions, finely chopped
3 garlic cloves, chopped
1 cup water
1 pound extra lean ground beef
½ pepper, chopped
15 ounces canned tomatoes
½ can condensed tomato soup
  (optional)

1 carrot, grated
1 stick celery, chopped
chopped mushrooms (optional)
2 bay leaves
oregano or marjoram
fresh parsley

Lightly cook onions and garlic with water in a large saucepan (no oil). Add mince and mix thoroughly with a fork to break up any lumps in the meat, then add remaining ingredients and simmer with the lid on for about 1 hour. Remove bay leaves and serve on pasta of your choice.

Serves 8 (130 cal/546 kJ per serve; with 1 cup pasta 330 cal/1386 kJ per serve).

POTATOES WITH SPINACH SAUCE

6 medium-sized scrubbed potatoes

SAUCE
1 dessertspoon olive oil
1 tablespoon wholemeal flour
2 garlic cloves, finely chopped
3 shallots, finely chopped

1 cup low-fat calcium-enriched milk or soy milk
6 large spinach leaves, steamed and blended to a smooth puree
1 tablespoon pine nuts
freshly ground black pepper

Prick holes in potatoes with a metal skewer to enable faster cooking. Dry bake in a moderate oven or microwave until cooked through. Slice thinly and arrange in a shallow dish.

Warm oil and mix in wholemeal flour, garlic and shallots. Stir over low heat for 1 minute. Add milk and continue stirring until mixture boils and thickens. Remove from heat and add pureed spinach, pine nuts and lots of black pepper. Pour over potatoes and serve immediately.

Serves 6 (approximately 155 cal/651 kJ per serve).

LOW-CALORIE CANNELLONI

½ pound cannelloni shells (uncooked)
* buy shells that do not need to be boiled first.

FILLING
6–8 spinach leaves, lightly steamed and roughly chopped
2–3 garlic cloves
1 onion, chopped
3 shallots and/or chives, chopped
½ cup chopped mushrooms
1 cup coarsely chopped ricotta cheese
⅓ cup crumbled fetta cheese

SAUCE
6 tomatoes, roughly chopped
2 shallots, finely chopped
1 small onion, finely chopped
½ pepper, chopped
1 tablespoon chopped fresh basil
1 tablespoon chopped fresh parsley
1 or 2 bay leaves

ALTERNATIVE CANNELLONI FILLING
6–8 spinach leaves, lightly steamed and chopped
2 carrots, grated
3 shallots and/or chives, finely chopped
1 dessertspoon chopped fresh dill
2 avocados, coarsely chopped
1 cup mung bean sprouts

Place all sauce ingredients in the microwave for 5–7 minutes or stir over moderate heat with no oil until cooked. (For your convenience you may wish to purchase a fresh napolitana sauce with similar ingredients and no added salt, preservatives or artificial additives from your local fruiterer, deli or supermarket.)

Combine all filling ingredients in blender and carefully fill cannelloni shells.

Line the base of a shallow rectangular dish with a third of the sauce. Carefully place a layer of filled cannelloni shells onto this, covering the entire base. Top with remaining sauce and bake in a moderate oven for approximately 40 minutes.

Serve with a large garden salad

Serves 7 (approximately 200 cal/840 kJ per serve; approximately 245 cal/1029 kJ per serve using alternative filling).

AVOCADO PASTA

3 avocados
6 garlic cloves
½ cup fresh basil
½ cup fresh parsley

⅓ cup pine nuts
freshly ground black pepper
juice of ½ lemon

Blend all ingredients together. Serve on hot cooked pasta of your choice, plus a garden salad.

Serves 6 (approximately 465 cal/1953 kJ per serve, including 1 cup pasta and garden salad.

EGGPLANT AND NAPOLITANA SAUCE FOR PASTA

> STEP TWO
> **MAINTENANCE**

2–3 eggplants
seasoned wholemeal flour
olive oil
wholemeal breadcrumbs
sesame seeds

NAPOLITANA SAUCE
2 cans peeled tomatoes or 8–10
   tomatoes, chopped
½ pepper, chopped
2 onions, chopped
handful of fresh chopped basil

Combine all sauce ingredients in saucepan and bring to the boil. Reduce heat and simmer for 30 minutes, stirring occasionally to prevent burning.

Wash and slice eggplants, sprinkle with salt and leave for 30 minutes. Place in large colander and rinse off salt under cold water. Pat dry and coat with seasoned flour.

Heat a little oil in a non-stick pan and lightly fry eggplant, being careful to drain well on absorbent paper.

Place a layer of eggplant in an ungreased casserole dish and top with a layer of basil sauce. Repeat this process using alternate layers of eggplant and sauce until all ingredients are used. Finish with a layer of sauce and sprinkle with wholemeal breadcrumbs and sesame seeds. Bake in a moderate oven for 20-30 minutes.

•*This is a delicious vegetable topping for pasta.*

Serves 6 (290 cal/1218 kJ per serve—excluding pasta).

BARBECUED MARINATED KING PRAWNS

STEP TWO
MAINTENANCE

12 green prawns or shrimp

MARINADE
2 tablespoons low-sodium soy
 sauce

1 inch ginger root, sliced
3 garlic cloves, finely chopped
2 fresh chillies, sliced
2 shallots, finely chopped
⅓ cup beer

Shell the prawns, removing heads but leaving the tails intact. Devein and wash the prawns under cold water.

Mix all the ingredients for the marinade together in a dish and place the prawns into this, making sure each prawn is coated with the mixture. Leave for at least 1 hour.

Strain off the liquid and cook the prawns, chilli, garlic, shallot and ginger on the barbecue until prawns change colour and are cooked through, about 7 to 10 minutes.

Serve with rice and salad.

Serves 4 (approximately 70 cal/294 kJ per serve).

DRY BEEF CURRY

STEP TWO
MAINTENANCE

3 pounds lean beef or trim lamb
1 tablespoon ground coriander
1 teaspoon ground cumin
¼ teaspoon ground cardamon
½ teaspoon cinnamon
½ teaspoon ground black pepper

1 medium onion
3 lime or lemon leaves
1 tablespoon fresh ginger root
3 garlic cloves
1 tablespoon rice flour
1 tablespoon lemon juice

Trim all visible fat from the meat and cut it into cubes. Combine all the dry herbs. Blend the onion, lime leaves, ginger, garlic, rice flour and lemon juice until smooth. Add the dry herbs and blend again making sure the mixture is well combined.

Mix the meat and curry paste together in a bowl, taking care to rub the paste well into the meat. Marinate for at least 1 hour (can be left overnight in the refrigerator).

The meat may then be threaded onto bamboo skewers and grilled or barbecued until tender.

Serve with rice and salad.

Serves 8 (approximately 400 cal/1680 kJ per serve).

CHINESE STIR-FRIED VEGETABLES

STEP TWO
MAINTENANCE

½ green pepper
½ red pepper
2 carrots
2 zucchinis
1 onion
4 shallots
1 head of broccoli
light olive oil
1 teaspoon sesame oil
1 tablespoon fish sauce
20 raw cashew nuts

2 garlic cloves, chopped
1 tablespoon chopped fresh ginger root
½ bunch fresh coriander, chopped
fresh chilli (optional)
freshly ground black pepper
2 tablespoons ketchup manis (sweet soy sauce from Asian shop)
4 tablespoons low-sodium soy sauce
1 small bunch spinach

Prepare the vegetables and cut into large bite-sized pieces. Wipe the wok or large pan with a cloth dipped in olive oil so the stir-fry will not stick (a non-stick pan is better because you need no oil). Place sesame oil and fish sauce into the wok with ¼ cup water, over a moderate–hot flame. Add the onion and cook until transparent. Then mix in the nuts, garlic, ginger and all the other vegetables except the spinach. Mix in the other sauces and more water if required, stirring constantly.

Break up the spinach leaves into small pieces and add just before the meal is ready to serve, as they require minimal cooking. All the vegetables should be slightly crunchy and the spinach should not lose its green color. Do not overcook.

Serve immediately with rice or noodles.

• *The addition of some sliced tofu (available at health food stores) to this dish will add more protein and calcium to this meal. Half a cup of tofu contains 130 mg of calcium.*

Serves 6 (approximately 120 cal/504 kJ per serve).

CHICK PEA CURRY

2 onions
1 stick lemon grass, finely chopped
5 garlic cloves
2 teaspoons grated ginger
¼ teaspoon fenugreek seeds
1 teaspoon turmeric
1 teaspoon dried chilli (optional)
1 teaspoon dried coriander
1 teaspoon cumin
½ teaspoon fennel seeds

6 cardamon pods
2 teaspoons paprika
1 cup of coconut milk or soy milk
2 cups pre-cooked chick peas
2 tablespoons vinegar
2 tomatoes, chopped
1 cinnamon stick
10 lime leaves
1 tablespoon low-sodium soy sauce

Blend together the onion, lemon grass, garlic and ginger to a paste. In a mortar and pestle grind together all the dry herbs and spices, except the cinnamon stick and lime leaves. Add the spices to the onion paste and continue to blend until they are also combined.

In a large saucepan place a tablespoon of the coconut milk and add curry paste to this. Cook over moderate heat for 5 minutes, stirring constantly. Add extra coconut milk, chick peas, vinegar, tomatoes, cinnamon, lime leaves and soy sauce. Simmer for half an hour, stirring occasionally.

Serves 4 (approximately 250 cal/1050 kJ per serve).

CARIBBEAN CHICKEN

2 pounds chicken thigh fillets, trimmed of fat
2 teaspoons paprika
2 garlic cloves, finely chopped

3 small dried chillies, finely chopped (optional)
3 tablespoons sweet mango chutney
½ cup coconut milk
2 tablespoons lime juice

Sprinkle chicken fillets with paprika and grill until golden. Transfer chicken to a casserole dish or saucepan. Combine all other ingredients in a bowl and mix well. Pour over chicken and cook over low to moderate heat for 25 minutes, turning chicken and stirring occasionally. The sauce will reduce and thicken.

When serving, spoon the sauce over the chicken.

Serves 8 (approximately 250 cal/1050 kJ per serve).

CHICKEN IN A PARCEL

STEP TWO
MAINTENANCE

2 chicken breasts
12 dried apricots, finely chopped
2 tablespoons low-fat yoghurt
2 tablespoons chopped walnuts
    or pecans

½ teaspoon thyme
freshly ground black pepper
8 sheets filo pastry plus extra
⅓ cup low-fat natural yoghurt
1-2 tablespoons olive oil
sesame seeds

Lightly pound chicken breasts to an even thickness. Cut in half. Combine apricots, yoghurt, nuts and spices together and spread evenly onto each piece. Roll up quickly.

Brush one sheet of filo with a little of the extra yoghurt and cover with a second sheet of pastry, brush again and fold in half to form a square. Place each chicken roll diagonally at the corner of a square of filo pastry, roll up into a pastry parcel, tucking the ends under as you go.

Place on a lightly greased baking tray and brush with a little olive oil. Sprinkle with sesame seeds and bake in a moderate oven for 35 minutes or until golden brown.

Serves 4 (350 cal/1470 kJ per serve).

TUNA BAKE

STEP TWO
MAINTENANCE

3 cups cooked brown rice
1 medium onion, chopped
2 sticks celery, chopped
Basic Foundation Sauce (recipe
    page 150)
3 shallots, chopped

½ cup corn kernels
18 ounces tuna in spring water,
    drained
1 handful of parsley, chopped
3 medium potatoes, cooked and
    mashed
breadcrumbs and a little parmesan
    cheese to sprinkle on top

Place rice in the base of a large casserole dish. Lightly cook onion and celery in a steamer or microwave to soften. Combine sauce, onion, celery, shallots, corn, tuna and parsley and mix well. Tip over the rice and top with the mashed potato. Sprinkle with some breadcrumbs and parmesan cheese. Bake in a moderate oven for half an hour.

Serves 4 (approximately 500 cal/2100 kJ per serve).

SALMON MORNAY

STEP TWO
MAINTENANCE

2 cups cooked pasta spirals
Mornay Sauce (recipe page 151)
½ pound pink salmon, drained
1 small onion, finely chopped
2 shallots, finely chopped
freshly ground black pepper

1 handful chopped
   fresh parsley
juice of 1 lemon
½ pepper, finely sliced
breadcrumbs and a little parmesan
   cheese for topping

Tip pasta into the base of a small casserole dish. Combine sauce, salmon, onion, shallots, pepper, parsley, lemon juice and pepper and tip over pasta. Sprinkle with breadcrumbs and parmesan and bake in a moderate oven for approximately half an hour.

Serves 4 (approximately 370 cal/1554 kJ per serve).

AUTHENTIC BOLOGNAISE SAUCE

STEP TWO
MAINTENANCE

2 pounds extra lean ground beef
2 small onions
½ bunch fresh basil
1 handful fresh Italian parsley
2 tablespoons olive oil (authentic
   recipe but is optional)
2 garlic cloves, finely chopped

30 ounces canned tomatoes
   or fresh equivalent, chopped
3¾ cups V8 Vegetable Juice
4 tablespoons tomato paste
1 bay leaf
freshly ground black pepper

In a large heavy-based saucepan, over low heat, brown the mince, squashing with a fork as you go to stop it forming lumps. Blend onions, basil and parsley with a blender, and add to mince, mixing well.

Next add oil and garlic, followed by tomatoes, V8 juice and tomato paste. Add bay leaf and pepper and cook over low heat, stirring occasionally and shaking the pot. Cook for 35–45 minutes.

Serves 8 (approximately 280 cal/1176 kJ per serve).

BLENDER CREPES

1 cup wholemeal flour
2 eggs
½ cup low-fat calcium-enriched
  milk or soy milk

⅓ cup water
1 tablespoon olive oil

Place ingredients in a blender in listed order. Blend for 30 seconds, stop and stir down sides. Blend for 1 minute until mixture is smooth. Cook in a non-stick frypan over moderate heat.

Makes 12 crepes (approximately 60 cal/252 kJ per serve).

•This is a slightly thick batter which, when cooked, is strong enough to hold fillings such as beef, chicken, rice or fish.

SAVOURY FILLINGS FOR CREPES

Make blender crepes. Use your imagination and fill each crepe with your own combinations of sauces, herbs, vegetables, meat, seafood, poultry or cooked legumes.

Try these combinations:

- Mushroom Sauce (recipe page 151), cooked brown rice, fresh tarragon, shallots and cubes of cooked chicken.

- Mornay Sauce (recipe page 151), cooked prawns, avocado and fresh parsley.

- lightly steamed vegetables with Dahl (recipe page 171) and raw cashews.

- Quick Mexican Beans (recipe page 171), Chilli Sauce (recipe page 149) and a little cottage cheese.

- Egg Sauce (recipe page 151), pureed spinach and fresh dill.

•Calories will differ according to amount of filling used. If low-fat fillings are used and you limit the serve size to 2 crepes per person, the caloric level will be suitable for STEP TWO—Maintenance Programme.

SWEET TREATS

WHOLEMEAL PANCAKES
1 cup soy milk or low fat
calcium-enriched milk
three quarter cup wholemeal
self raising flour
1 egg
1 teaspoon vanilla essence

Beat egg with half the milk. Mix in half the flour, then the rest of the milk and flour alternately. Beat well, making sure there are no lumps. Add the vanilla essence and let the mixutre stand for 15 minutes.

Prepare a pan by brushing with oil, otherwise use a non-stick pan.

Over a moderate heat, pour approximately one quarter of a cup of mixture into the pan. Pancakaes are ready to turn when bubbles appear over top surface. Turn once and serve when cooked through.

Makes 6-8 pancakes (approximately 90cal/378 kJ per serve.)

APPLE AND OATBRAN MUFFINS
1 large apple, grated
1¼ cups rolled oats
1 ¼ cup oatbran
2 tablespoons olive oil
¼ cup raisins
1 tablespoon chopped walnuts
poppy seeds

Combine all ingredients, except poppy seeds, in a large bowl and mix well. Spoon into non-stick muffin pans and sprinkle with poppy seeds. Bake in a moderate oven 350° F for 25 minutes.

Makes 8 muffins (approximately 160 cal/672 kJ each).

BANANA AND PECAN MUFFINS

2 medium bananas, mashed
2 tablespoons honey
2 tablespoons olive oil
½ teaspoon vannilla essence

1¼ cups wholemeal self-raising flour
1 tablespoon chopped pecan nuts
sesame seeds

Mix bananas, honey and oil in a large bowl. Fold in remaining ingredients, except sesame seeds and mix lightly. Spoon into non stick muffin pans and sprinkle with sesame seeds. Bake in a moderate oven 350° F for approximately 20 minutes.
Makes 8 muffins (approx 170/cal/714 kJ each).

BLUEBERRY MUFFINS

½ cup low-fat calcium-enriched milk
¼ cup ricotta cheese
2 eggs
3 tablespoons olive oil

2 cups wholemeal self-raising flour
½ cup oatbran
1 tablespoon sugar
1½ punnet blueberries

Blend together the milk, ricotta cheese and eggs, then add oil to this mixture then blend again.
Combine the dry ingredients together in a large bowl. Make a well in the centre, pour in the blended mixture and mix well.
Lastly, fold through the fresh blueberries. Spoon into a non-stick muffin pan and bake in a moderate oven 350° F for 25 minutes or until golden brown.

Makes 18 (approximately 100 cal/420 kJ per muffin).

BANANA CREAM

Peel and freeze ripe or overripe bananas.

When bananas are frozen solid, blend them well with a blender. The mixture becomes thick and creamy, resembling banana ice cream.

• *Bananas are rich in potassium which is necessary for cellular and enzyme activity.*

Each medium-sized banana yields 90 cal/378 kJ.

ICED MANGO TREAT

Freeze rip or overripe mango pulp
1 egg white per cup of mango pulp

When the mango pulp is frozen solid, blend with some egg white using a blender. Serve while mango still contains some ice crystals.

•This is delicious on a hot day after a meal to clean the palate. It is low in calories and rich in vitamins C and A.

Approximately 120cal/504 kJ per mango.

BERRY DELICIOUS

1 cup of raspberries or berries
of your choice
1 tablespoon honey
juice of 1 orange

2 teaspoons gelatine
One cup part skim ricotta cheese
Extra fresh berries and mint to garnish

Heat raspberries, honey and orange juice together until hot, but not boiling. Dissolve gelatine in a little hot water and mix through. Blend lightly with ricotta cheese and place into individual serving dishes. Garnish with extra berries and mint.

Serves 4 (approx 160 cal/672 kJ per serve).

MINTED PINEAPPLE SORBET

1 cup water
1 cup unsweetened pineapple juice
1 tablespoon chopped mint
¼ cup castor sugar

1 tablespoon lemon lime juice
1 cup blended fresh pineapple
2 egg whites

Combine water, juice, mint and sugar and boil for three minutes. Set aside to cool. When cool add lemon juice and blended pineapple and mix well. Place in a freezer tray and partially freeze.

Whip egg whites into a meringue and fold through pineapple mixture. Refreeze.

Serves 8 (165 cal/693 kJ per serve).

BAKED RICE PUDDING

STEP TWO
MAINTENANCE

½ cup brown rice
2½ cups soy milk
1 egg, beaten

2 teaspoons golden syrup
2 teaspoon grated lemon rind
grated nutmeg

Soak rice in soy milk for half an hour in a small ovenproof dish. Mix in egg, syrup and rind. Sprinkle with grated nutmeg and bake in a slow oven 250° F to 300° F for 2½ hours, stir after 30 mintues.

Serves 4 (approxiamately 120 cal/504 kJ per serve.)

PASSIONFRUIT AND ROCKMELON MOUSSE

STEP TWO
MAINTENANCE

3 teaspoons gelatine
½ cup hot water
1 rockmelon, roughly chopped
¼ cup loosely packed brown sugar
(optional)

½ cup orange juice
4 medium passionfruit

Sprinkle gelatine into hot water and stir with a fork until dissolved. Add water and gelatine to rockmelon, sugar and orange juice and blend until smooth and frothy.
Gently fold through passionfruit pulp and pour into one large bowl or four individual bowls. Refrigerate until partially set, stir again, then return mousse to refrigerator until set.

Serves 4 (125 cal/525kJ/serve or 88 cal/370 kJ without sugar).

•*Rich in Vitamin C and fiber this is a delicious option if you are craving sweets. If you serve it with a dessertspoon of low-fat yoghurt you only add about 30 calories and you increase your daily calcium intake by 100 mg.*

FRESH FRUIT SORBET

2 cups strawberries
1 tablespoon lime or lemon juice
2 egg whites

¼ cup castor sugar

Blend strawberries with lime or lemon juice and pour into freezer tray. Partially freeze until ice crystals start to form.
Whip egg whites and sugar until mixture forms peaks, and fold through fruit mixture. Refreeze until set.

• *The addition of citrus in this recipe makes it tangy and refreshing to the palate. Count this as a daily fruit serving. Other fruits such as paw paw, mango, melons and berries can be used in this recipe.*

4 Serves: 55cal/231 kJ per serve; 6 Serves: 35 cal/147 kJ per serve.

LEMON SELF SAUCING PUDDING

1 tablespoon olive oil
1/3 cup sugar
2 eggs
2 level tablespoons wholemeal
self raising flour

2 teaspoons grated lemon rind
juice from 1 large or 2 small
lemons
1 cup low-fat calcium-enriched
milk or soy milk

Mix olive oil with sugar. Separate white from yolks of eggs. Add the flour to the oil and sugar. Add grated lemon rind, juice, yolks and milk; mix well. Beat egg whites to a merangue, and fold through mixture.
Pour into a lightly greased small casserole dish. Stand this in a baking dish containing cold water.
Bake in moderate oven for 40 minutes.

4 Serves: 55cal/231 kJ per serve; 6 Serves: 35 cal/147 kJ per serve.

APPLE CRUMBLE

STEP TWO
MAINTENANCE

4 green cooking apples
½ teaspoon allspice
½ tablespoon sugar or honey
2 tablespoons water

CRUMBLE MIX
2 tablespoons rolled oats
1 tablespoon dessicated coconut
1 tablespoon wholemeal flour
2 teaspoons sugar
2 tablespoons low-fat yoghurt

Peel, core and quarter the apples and stew them with the spice, sugar and water until just cooked. Place them in an ovenproof dish. In a small bowl mix the dry crumble mix ingredients together and add just enough yoghurt to bind the mixture together. Mixture should still be quite dry. Sprinkle evenly over the top of the apples and bake in a moderate oven without a lid until crumbles turns golden brown, about 20-30 minutes.

Serves 4 (approx 125 cal/525 kJ per serve).

CREAMY ALMOND FLUMMERY

STEP TWO
MAINTENANCE

3/4 cup cold water
1/3 cup brown sugar
3 teaspoons gelatine
3/4 cup boiling water
1 ¼ cups low fat evaporated milk or soy milk

almond essence to taste
slivered toasted almonds
1 piece of glace ginger, finely chopped to garnish

Place cold water in dish and add sugar. Sprinkle gelatine on top and stir in as you add boiling water. Keep stirring until gelatine and sugar have dissolved. Add milk and almond essence, mix throughly. Pour into a medium serving bowl or 4 individual dishes. Garnish with almonds and ginger. Chill until firm.

Serves 4 (if evaporated milk used, 110 cal/462 kJ per serve, if soy milk 150 cal/630 kJ per serve).

POACHED PEARS

STEP TWO
MAINTENANCE

3 pears, peeled, halved and cored
½ cup water
½ cup pear juice (apple or
orange may be used)

1 inch cinnamon stick
2 broken cardamon pods
(optional)
1 crushed vanilla bean (optional)

Place all ingredients except pears, in large pan and simmer gently for 10 minutes. Add pears and cook until soft, do not overcook. Remove cinnamon stick, cardamon and vanilla bean. Serve with Vanilla Yoghurt Sauce (recipe page 190) or Almond Custard Cream (recipe below.) An alternative would be to use 1 teaspoon of rose water instead of the other spices.

• This recipe could also be made in the microwave and the pears filled with spoonfuls of a mixture of chopped prunes, ginger powder, chopped almonds or pecans and brown sugar.

Serves 6 (100 cal/420 kJ serve, including filling).

ALMOND CUSTARD CREAM

STEP TWO
MAINTENANCE

1 egg
2 teaspoons honey
1 cup low-fat calcium-enriched
milk or soy milk

1 teaspoon cornflour
1 teaspoon almond essence

Beat egg and honey together until well combined. Save a little milk to combine with cornflour and heat remainder of milk over moderate heat until lukewarm. Add honey and egg, stirring well. Blend cornflour with a little milk and add to other ingredients. Stir constantly until mixture boils and thickens. It should be the consistency of a thin custard. Remove from heat and add almond essence.
Serve hot or clod.

Serves 4 (65-75 cal/250 kJ per serve).

FLAPJACKS

STEP TWO
MAINTENANCE

2 eggs
2 tablespoons brown sugar
4 tablespoons LSA (see pg 209)
½ cup water

1 cup wholemeal self-raising
 flour
1½ cups low- fat calcium-
 enriched
 milk or soy milk

Beat egg with the brown sugar and add LSA and water, mix well. Fold in ½ cup of flour, then ½ cup of milk. Mix in remaining flour followed by the rest of the milk. Let stand for half an hour to thicken.

Cook tablespoonfuls in a non-stick pan, turn once when bubbles appear on top. The LSA contains linseed oil, so you will find the more flapjacks you cook, the easier they are to turn.

•This recipe is rich in fiber, protein and calcium. Serve flapjacks hot or cold with fresh fruit and yoghurt toppings.

Makes 24 flapjacks (approx 50 cal/210 kJ each).

TOPPINGS

VANILLA YOGHURT SAUCE

STEP TWO
MAINTENANCE

1 egg, separated
1 tablespoon honey
1 cup low-fat acidophilus yoghurt

½ teaspoon vanilla
cinnamon or nutmeg if desired

Combine egg yolk, honey ,yoghurt, vanilla and spice and mix well. Beat egg white until stiff and fold through youghurt mixture. Serve fresh, this mixture will not keep.

Serves 4 (75 cal/315 kJ per serve).

FRESH PAPAYA SAUCE

pulp of ½ papaya (pawpaw)
1 dessertspoon lime or lemon juice
1 teaspoon grated lemon rind

½ cup low-fat natural yoghurt
½ teaspoon ginger powder

Blend ingredients until smooth and serve immediately.

•*This sauce is easily digested because it is rich in enzymes. It is an excellent source of vitamin C, vitamin A and calcium*

Serves 4 (30 cal/126 kJ per serve).

EATING TIPS THAT CAN SAVE YOUR LIFE

There is so much information available today that many women are confused when making decisions about their dietary needs.

This section will explain how to use your food as a healing tool. You can allow your food to be your medicine and by following my recommendations and adopting good eating habits, you are preventing illness and improving vitality, health and well-being.

I have done a great deal of research into this subject so I have included the latest breakthroughs and vital facts on nutrition, that every woman, desirous of good health for herself and her family, must know.

CARBOHYDRATES

Carbohydrate foods have a very important role in your diet. They are nutritious and filling and are excellent foods for achieving successful weight loss.

The main carbohydrates present in foods are sugars, starches and cellulose. The sugars and starches are converted by enzymes in your digestive juices to **glucose**, your blood sugar. This is your primary energy source. The cellulose contributes very little energy but provides you with bulk and fiber for intestinal motility and improves elimination.

Some of your glucose is converted to **glycogen** and stored in your muscle tissue and your liver. When your blood-sugar level is low, glucose can be released back into the bloodstream to provide you with the energy you need.

> **The best sources of carbohydrates in your diet are wholemeal breads and crackers, cereals and grains, legumes (dried peas, lentils and beans), nuts and seeds, pasta, starchy vegetables and fruits.**

They are more accurately called **complex carbohydrates**. This is because they have a complex molecular structure. **They are full of nutrients and are naturally low in fat.**

Complex carbohydrates are more satisfying because they usually require more chewing and therefore take longer to eat. They provide you with a slower release of energy over a longer period of time, which is great for people who are trying to lose weight.

By eating a diet which is high in complex carbohydrates you will not have the 'highs and lows' associated with fluctuating blood-sugar levels. This will also reduce your cravings for sweets.

> **Keeping a high level of complex carbohydrates in your diet and doing regular exercise, will burn fat and will achieve healthier weight loss.**

Diets low in complex carbohydrate cause us to lose weight quickly by the loss of fluid and lean muscle tissue. As soon as we break our diet the weight comes straight back. We need our lean muscle tissue to keep us firm, not flabby and to support our skeleton. Good muscle tone means less lower back and neck problems.

The unhealthy sugars and starches are refined carbohydrates. These provide fast energy and usually no nutrients. Refined carbohydrates are polished rice, white sugar, white flour and products made from these such as cakes, biscuits, sweets and white bread. When you eat these foods you get a sudden rise in blood sugar, followed by a rapid drop. This leaves you craving more sweets and can often cause fatigue, headache, nervousness and giddiness.

> Research shows that a diet high in complex carbohydrates will protect you against many illness, including obesity, cancer, diabetes and heart disease.

By following our Body Shaping Diet you will ensure that your diet is rich in healthy complex carbohydrates. You will achieve weight loss without losing energy and you will burn fat not muscle tissue.

BREAD AND CRACKERS

While you are on the Body Shaping Diet weight loss programme—**STEP ONE**, I recommend that you have **three servings each day** from this food group. I have included a short list of desirable bread and crackers from which you may select freely. **If you do not have cereal for breakfast then you may increase your allowance to four serves.**

I recommend wholemeal choices as this is the best way to increase your daily fiber intake. You will also boost your nutritional input because the outside husk of the grain contains those essential B group vitamins for a healthy nervous system. This part of the grain also contains zinc which improves your memory and maintains healthy hair, skin and nails.

White flour products only provide you with starch which gives you temporary energy and a feeling of fullness.

When selecting bread try to avoid loaves made with baker's or breadmaking flour. It tends to have very low levels of zinc and high levels of cadmium, which is a toxic trace mineral that can increase hypertension.

If you don't like the heavy grain bread then simply choose a lighter wholemeal or stoneground loaf. Try not to limit yourself to wheatbread alone. There are some delicious loaves available made from rye, barley, corn and oats, to name a few.

If you would like to avoid yeast in bread then try a sourdough loaf, or yeast-free pita bread.

You and your family will all benefit from the added fiber and nutrition.

Select three or four servings per day from the list below.
1 SERVING = APPROXIMATELY 75 CAL/315 kJ

1 slice wholemeal bread
½ bread roll
1 slice pumpernickel
½ wholemeal muffin
½ pita bread
4 Finn Crisp
2 WASA multigrain crispbread
2 Ryvita crackers with sesame
3 wholemeal Saltine crackers
4 rice crispbreads
2 rice cakes
8 rice crackers (unsalted)
1 large taco shell
½ wholemeal scone
1 small wholemeal pancake

On our Maintenance Programme—**STEP TWO**, you will increase your bread intake by one more serve. This means you will have four serves each day from this group plus cereal.

CEREAL CHOICES

When you are selecting a breakfast cereal, take the time to read the product information on the packaging. You may be surprised to find that some popular brands have extremely high levels of fat, sodium and sugar.

I recommend that you choose from the following list.

¾ cup oatmeal	100 cal/420 kJ
½ cup barley	110 cal/462 kJ
½ cup brown rice	120 cal/504 kJ
2 Weetabix	94 cal/395 kJ
2 Granose	96 cal/403 kJ
1 ounce Kellogg's Low Fat Granola	120 cal/504 kJ
1 ounce Quaker 100% Low Fat	110 cal/462 kJ
1 ounce Just Right	108 cal/450 kJ
1 ounce Balance	117 cal/490 kJ
1 ounce Low Fat Alpen	110 cal/462 kJ
1 ounce Komplete Natural Muesli	111 cal/469 kJ
1 ounce Familia No Added SugarMuesli	95 cal/400 kJ
1 ounce Kölln Crispy Oats	100 cal/420 kJ
1 ounce Kölln Crispy Oats	110 cal/462 kJ
1 ounce Fruit & Fiber Cereal	108 cal/450 kJ

MILK AND CALCIUM REQUIREMENTS

Generally speaking, women require 800–1000 mg of calcium daily. During pregnancy, lactation and menopause our calcium needs increase to 1100–1200 mg per day.

Every woman should check that her daily diet provides these amounts of calcium (see table page 196).

If your diet on any one day falls short of this, or if you are not sure, take a **good quality** calcium tablet containing 600 mg of calcium every day.

One of the highest sources of calcium is milk and you will see from the calcium table on page 196 that a cup of milk daily will give you a good start to meeting your daily requirements. If you are following a Dairy Free diet and cannot drink cows' milk, you may choose soy milk and oat or rice milk products instead. These are good low-calorie alternatives but contain small amounts of calcium.

GOOD CALCIUM FOODS

FOOD	AVERAGE SERVE	MILLIGRAMS OF CALCIUM
Whole milk	1 cup	300
Skim milk	1 cup	408
Lactaid non fat milk, calcium fortified	1 cup	500
Easylac non fat milk	1 cup	300
Nonfat buttermilk	1 cup	300
Goats' milk	1 cup	295
Creamy Original Vitasoy	1 cup	80
Rice milk	1 cup	2.5
Soy milk (unfortified)	1 cup	60
Soy milk (fortified)	1 cup	300
Powdered skim milk	1 tablespoon	130
Hi Calcium Borden	1 cup	1,000
VIVA (with extra calcium)	1 cup	500
Plain nonfat yogurt/ plain low-fat yogurt	6 to 8 ounces	240
Farmer or pot cheese	1 ounce	258
Feta cheese	1 ounce	129
Low-fat cottage cheese	1 ounce	35
Ricotta cheese	1 ounce	100
Egg (Large)	2 ounces	35
Sardines	3.5 ounces	350
Salmon	3.5 ounces	190
Tuna (with bones)	3.5 ounces	290
Fish (fresh, cooked)	3.5 ounces	35
Almonds (unsalted)	1 ounce (25 nuts/average)	70
Brazil nuts (unsalted)	1 ounce (7–8 nuts)	55
Walnuts (unsalted)	1 ounce (25 nuts/average)	30
Pistachio nuts (unsalted)	1 ounce (23 nuts/average)	40
Whole sesame seeds	1 ounce (2½ tablespoons)	290
Sunflower seeds	1 ounce (2½ tablespoons)	30
Rhubarb	half cup (cooked)	170
Orange	1	50
Rockmelon (cantaloupe)	half	30
Fresh fruit	each piece (average)	10–30
Brocolli	1 cup	50
Spinach	1cup	100
Vegetables	1 cup (average)	10–50
Chick peas	½ cup	75
Baked beans	½ cup	60
Kidney beans	½ cup	60
Soy beans	½ cup	90
Bread (average all types)	1 slice	30
Cereal (average all types)	1 ounce	5–30
Tahini (sesame paste)	1 tablespoon	85
Hummus	1 tablespoon	15
Tofu	½ cup	130

You will see in the calcium table that some good soy milks, unfortunately, are not a good source of calcium. Therefore you will need to make sure your diet is supplemented with other foods rich in calcium or take a calcium tablet on retiring at night.

When choosing soy milk remember to carefully read the contents of the milk on the packaging. Some soy products are high in sugar to make them more palatable. You can buy low-fat varieties of soy milk if you wish. I use soy in recipes as a substitute for cream or to give a creamy texture to sauces, soups or custards.

Rice milk is a low-calorie beverage and is a delicious and refreshing drink, however it is low in calcium.

If you drink cows' milk then I recommend calcium-enriched milk, which is low in fat and much higher in calcium than skim milk.

SUGAR

While you are on **STEP ONE** of the Body Shaping diet it is generally a good idea to avoid sugar that doesn't occur naturally in your food. The addition of sugar can quickly add unnecessary calories and it is easy to consume large amounts. One teaspoon of sugar contains about 20 cal/84 kJ and it has no essential nutrients. It doesn't satisfy your hunger and, in fact, once you start on sugar you may find that you will binge all day. This is particularly true for the gynaeoid and thyroid body shapes.

Watch labels for high-sugar levels in convenience foods such as soy milk, bottled sauces, spreads and canned foods. Remember that ingredients are listed in decreasing order of weight, so if sugar is listed first on the label then that food is chiefly made up of sugar. All ingredients ending in the suffix 'ose' are sugars. Examples to watch for are sucrose, lactose, fructose, maltose and glucose. Other sugars are sorbitol and mannitol.

The difference between brown or black sugar, and raw or white sugar, is simply that it is less refined.

Molasses is a by-product of sugar refining and is the best choice of sweetener because it has slightly less calories than other sugars and the benefit of added nutrients, namely iron, calcium and potassium.

Honey is a very natural and pure product, however it does contain the same amount of calories as crystal sugar. The benefit of honey over sugar is that you tend to use less of it.

> When you have a craving for sweets try to satisfy it with small amounts of wholegrain foods or fruit. This will be more satisfying and will stabilize your blood-sugar level, eliminating the urge for sweets.

Sometimes cravings for sweet foods can be overwhelming. The supplements on page 75 can reduce or prevent cravings for sugar and chocolates.

> It can be difficult to satisfy a craving for chocolate with a bowl of rice. Chances are that you are looking for comfort food rather than experiencing blood-sugar fluctuations.
>
> Try having a cup of hot cocoa or carob (not hot chocolate), made with skim or soy milk and sweetened with a little honey, molasses or brown sugar. By doing this you will satisfy the chocolate urge without all the added caffeine and fat.

ARTIFICIAL SWEETENERS

Artificial sweeteners are generally best avoided. They are chemically made and long-term effects on health are still unknown.

Aspartame is a chemical found in some artificial sweeteners that can affect your nervous system by interfering with your ability to relax. **Aspartame is broken down into formaldehyde and methanol and these are highly toxic. See www.dorway.com.** Watch for hidden sodium in artificial sweeteners.

I do realise though, that you may enjoy a soft drink occasionally or wish to make a sweet that is not going to add unwanted calories. In this case you should go ahead and not feel guilty about doing so.

THE SUGAR–FAT CONNECTION

Many overweight women do not like sugar alone, however research has shown that when sugar is combined with cream, milk or fat, they love it.

Android-shaped women often tell me that if cakes and pastries are available to them, they will eat them, even though they don't necessarily enjoy them.

Sweet foods tend to be rich in fat and this is where the danger lurks. **Sugar makes fat more palatable and when it is added to high-fat foods it encourages the obese to consume more.**

Foods rich in sugar and fat will often replace nutritional foods in our diet, which can lead to vitamin and mineral deficiency.

If you are feeling like icecream then have sorbet made from fresh fruit, water-based gelati or tofu icecream instead. They still contain sugar but it comes without the fat.

PROTEINS

Proteins are present in every cell of our bodies and are an important element in the growth, health and repair of all body tissues. This includes skin, hair, nails, internal organs, bones, cartilage, muscle tissue and blood.

They are also needed to manufacture hormones, enzymes for proper digestion and antibodies to fight infection.

During digestion, proteins within our food are broken down into simpler particles called amino acids. The amino acids are like building blocks which link together to form 'human' protein, which can be used within our bodies.

Some amino acids are not manufactured by our bodies and must be provided in our foods. They are called the essential amino acids. They must all be present together, in the correct proportions, in order for our protein to be utilized.

Some foods meet our needs perfectly. We call them **complete protein** foods. They are mainly animal products such as meat, fish, poultry, eggs, milk and cheese. Soy beans are also a good source of protein and contain many of the essential amino acids.

Foods which lack any one of the essential amino acids are called **incomplete proteins**. They are from plant sources and need to be combined in a meal to make sure you have the correct balance of amino acids.

Incomplete protein foods are grains, nuts, seeds, legumes (dried peas and beans), lentils, cereal, rice and pasta.

Combining protein is not difficult and it is very easy and safe to follow a vegetarian diet. It simply means that you would choose more than one food from this incomplete protein group with each meal.

So instead of having just lentils and vegetable, you would have lentils, brown rice and vegetable. Some other examples are:

Cereal with soy milk or low-fat milk.
Baked beans and wholemeal toast.
Pasta with pesto sauce (contains pine nuts)
Tahini on wholemeal bread.
Brown rice with lentils.
Legumes with brown rice.
Chickpeas with tahini (as in Hummus, recipe page 154).

Some ready made products which are good protein foods are hummus, falafel, tofu, tempeh and other soy products.

Adding some soy, dairy products or eggs into your diet makes it easier to have the correct balance of amino acids. However if you follow a strict vegetarian diet you will need to take care with combinations.

> **If you are a meat eater, as a general rule, try to get two-thirds of your protein from plants and only one-third from animal sources.**

PROTEIN REQUIREMENTS

Women require about 1.6 ounces (45g) of protein daily. This will alter slightly between the different body shapes. By following the eating plans in this book you will be having the correct amount of protein for your body type.

Remember that your daily protein intake must be increased during adolescence, pregnancy and lactation and be guided by your doctor or dietician during these times.

Here is a short list giving examples of protein levels in food.

3.5 ounces meat, poultry cooked	= 30 g protein
3.5 ounces tuna	= 29 g protein
3.5 ounces salmon	= 20 g protein
1 egg	= 6 g protein
1 cup low-fat calcium-enriched milk	= 12 g protein
1 cup soy milk	= 8 g protein
1 cup plain yoghurt	= 8 g protein
½ cup baked beans	= 8 g protein
½ cup brown rice	= 3 g protein
½ cup soy beans	= 13 g protein
2 Weetbix	= 4 g protein
¾ cup cooked oats	= 3 g protein
1 slice wholemeal bread	= 3 g protein

> **Try to obtain regular protein from plant and fish sources, not just land animals. This alone will ensure a low cholesterol level and a reduction in fats. Plant sources also provide us with additional carbohydrate and fiber.**

HIGH-PROTEIN DIETS

When we eat more protein than we need, we store most of the excess as fat. The rest is converted to nitrogen and is flushed out of the body in the urine. As a result your urine can be loaded with ammonia and other toxic by-products. This can place unnecessary strain on the kidneys.

Research has shown that eating excessive amounts of protein has been linked to kidney disease, osteoporosis, heart disease and cancer.

> Many athletes are led to believe that high-protein diets are best for them. This is not so. They need a diet rich in complex carbohydrates so their muscles are rich in glycogen. This will maintain a steady release of energy for stamina and endurance.

Don't forget, excess protein is not turned into muscle, it is turned into fat!

LEGUMES

Legumes include many varieties of lentils, peas and beans, such as red or brown lentils, chick peas, black-eyed peas, pinto beans, navy beans, soy beans, borlotti beans, red kidney beans, canellini beans and more. **They are all low in fat and rich in fiber, protein and carbohydrate, which make them an excellent substitute for meat in your diet.** All you have to remember is that some are incomplete proteins and as such need to be combined with other complementary protein foods.

For example, if you have a chick pea casserole, you would serve it with brown rice. A taco mixture made from kidney beans could be served with some natural yoghurt. Lentil burgers can be rolled in sesame seeds and served on a wholemeal bread roll.

> **When you combine legumes with nuts, seeds, grains, cereal or dairy products you can be sure that your protein and nutritional needs are met.**

Adding legumes to meat dishes will extend the meal, add fiber and improve its nutritional value.

Legumes are an economical food and they contain iron, thiamine (B1), riboflavin (B2) and niacin (B3). When they are sprouted, they are also an excellent source of vitamin C.

HOW TO COOK LEGUMES

Rinse the dried beans and place them in a large bowl with water (one cup beans to three cups water). Cover with a tea-towel or cloth and soak overnight.

Another quicker method is to cover the beans with water and bring them to the boil. Boil for two minutes and remove from heat. Cover and leave for one hour.

Soaking will retain the moisture that has been lost in the drying process. Unsoaked beans will be difficult to digest.

Brown lentils are much smaller than other legumes and only require minimal soaking.

Rinse the beans and place them in a saucepan of boiling water. You may wish to add some herbs, garlic or chopped onion to the water to add extra flavour. Do not add salt as this will make the beans tough. Reduce heat and simmer for thirty minutes or until the beans are soft and plump. Old beans will take longer to cook. Drain the beans and proceed with the recipe.

If you are making a casserole, you can mix the presoaked beans directly into the dish, adding extra water or stock as required.

For convenience you may prefer to use canned beans. These have been prepared for you and require no soaking or precooking. Drain off their liquid and add these directly to your recipe.

FRUIT

People on weight-reducing diets must be careful to select foods which are high in nutritional value and not high in calories. Fruit is an excellent choice, providing us with essential vitamins, minerals and fiber.

Some fruits such as pineapple and pawpaw, are rich in enzymes which assist our digestion and can help us absorb other nutrients. For example, if you wish to absorb more iron from your food then simply serve the meal with fruit rich in vitamin C such as pawpaw, pineapple or citrus.

Always try to have fresh fruit which is in season. Juices are fine but often the pulp is left behind and this is needed to provide extra fiber. Whole fruit is more satisfying. You will be more likely to remain hungry if you just drink the juice.

The skin and white pith of citrus and some other fruits contain the bioflavanoids or vitamin P. They are essential for the proper absorption of vitamin C. They keep collagen (our intercellular ce-

ment) in a healthy condition and strengthen our blood capillaries. This prevents haemorrhages, rupture of veins, bruising and slows down the ageing process. Rutin is part of the bioflavanoids and is essential in the prevention and treatment of varicose conditions. Including this nutrient in your diet often eliminates tired aching legs. Simply grate some of the rind when making citrus juices and add it to the drink.

If you cannot get fresh fruit, the next best choice would be frozen fruit followed by canned fruit in natural fruit juice. Dried fruits do not contain added sugar, however they may have a preservative added to maintain the nutrients and some people may be sensitive to this. Dried fruits can also harbor molds, which need to be avoided if you have problems with allergies, vaginal thrush or candida. Remember that dried fruits have simply had the water removed so they are equal in calories to fresh fruit and it is easy to eat too many.

> If you have problems with blood-sugar levels then eat your fruit with natural yoghurt or nuts and seeds. You will find that this will sustain your blood sugar for a longer period and provide a sense of fullness.

A lack of fruit in the diet will lead to serious health problems. **Fruit is rich in nutrients and I recommend three to five serves of fruit daily.** Try not to exceed this amount.

Keep in mind that you must watch your intake of all foods, even the 'healthy' ones. This is clear when we remind ourselves that cows can get fat by eating only grass.

FRUIT SERVINGS

While on the Body Shaping Weight Loss Diet—**STEP ONE**, I recommend that you have only **three serves of fruit** each day.

When you move to the Maintenance Programme—**STEP TWO**, you are allowed **five serves of fruit** each day.

EACH ONE OF THE FOLLOWING = 50–70 CAL/250kJ = 1 FRUIT SERVE

½ cup fresh fruit salad
½ medium to large banana
⅓ babaco
1 small apple or 4 ounces apple juice
2 kiwifruit
½ small pawpaw
½ rockmelon/honeydew
½ large pear
¾ cup raw berries
20 small cherries
⅓ custard apple
1 large fig
½ large grapefruit or 4 ounces unsweetened juice
small bunch grapes or 2.5 ounces grape juice
1 medium guava
6 small limes
3 small lemons
12 loquats
20 longan
6 lychees
1 large or 2 small mandarins

½ large or 1 small mango
1 medium nashi fruit
1½ pepino
1 medium orange or 4 ounces fresh juice
3 small passionfruit
1 medium peach/nectarine
2 small slices fresh pineapple
2 small plums
6 rambutans
2 starfruit (carambola)
1 cup strawberries
1½ tamarillo
1 cup watermelon balls
1 small persimmon
1½ pomelo
1½ quince
5–6 medium kumquats
2.5 ounces jackfruit
2 ounces durian
3 fresh apricots
2 large pomegranate
½ cup canned fruit in natural juice

DRIED FRUIT SERVINGS EACH ONE OF THE FOLLOWING = 1 FRUIT SERVE = 50–70 CAL/250 kJ

6 pieces apple
4 pieces apricot
1½ tablespoons
   currants/raisins/sultanas
3 pitted dates
1½ figs
4 prunes

3 strips mango
1½ tablespoons mixed fruit peel
1 ounce papaya spears
1 ounce peach
3/4 ounce pear
3/4 ounce pineapple

VEGETABLES

Fresh vegetables are a rich source of nutrients and fiber and contain no fat. Starchy vegetables like potato, sweet potato, carrots and beet are also a good source of carbohydrate to boost your energy levels and potassium which regulates your fluid balance. Do not omit these vegetables in order to cut calories. **They are packed full of vitamins and minerals and are only fattening if they are cooked in fat or oil.**

> **The Body Shaping Diet allows you to have unlimited green vegetables and salad. This is because they are low in calories and will actually speed your weight loss.**

Watery green vegetables assist the digestion of other foods. Meat and dairy products are heavy foods that tend to move through your intestines slowly. The addition of green vegetables will add water, fiber and enzymes to improve your ability to break down these foods and speed their elimination.

Green vegetables are extremely rich in the B group vitamins. These are water soluble and vital in the breakdown of fats and proper functioning of your nervous system.

> **Some B vitamins are destroyed at boiling point and for this reason green vegetables must be eaten raw or steamed to retain these important nutrients. Take care if you microwave green vegetables that you do not exceed boiling point.**

Yellow vegetables are an excellent source of vitamin A, a fat-soluble vitamin. Examples are: carrots, sweet potato, pumpkin, parsnip, turnip and squash. Spinach, broccoli and beet greens also contain large amounts of vitamin A.

This vitamin maintains the health of your skin and the soft tissue that lines your digestive tract, kidneys and bladder. It reduces your susceptibility to infection and inflammation in these areas. Vitamin A also assists your eyesight and the health of your lungs, mouth, nose, throat and sinuses.

Cooking, mashing or pureeing yellow vegetables helps to release vitamin A from the cell membranes. It is more difficult to absorb and utilise this nutrient from raw food.

Vegetables which contain water-soluble vitamins are sensitive to cooking, whereas vegetables that contain fat-soluble vitamins need to be cooked to release the nutrients. This explains the importance of eating a **balance of raw and cooked food** in your diet.

For optimum nutrition choose fresh vegetables as your first choice, frozen vegetables next and canned vegetables last.

The best vegetables will be those that have been grown organically, picked ripe and eaten while still fresh.

FIBER

Some fiber is rough and visible like the husk around grain or the skin on fruit. We call this **insoluble fiber** because it will not dissolve. During digestion we cannot break it down with enzymes or gastric secretions. Instead it absorbs water and provides bulk to our faeces. Our stools become softer and heavier, which allows them to move through our intestines faster. As a result we eliminate constipation and reduce the incidence of diverticulitis, appendicitis, bowel cancer, spastic colon, hemorrhoids and other varicose conditions.

Other types of plant fiber may consist of gums, pectin and mucilages and this is called **soluble fiber.** It dissolves easily in water and is found in legumes, cereal, oatbran, fruits and vegetables. This soluble fiber protects us against gall stones, ulcerative colitis, Crohns disease, high blood pressure, high blood cholesterol and diabetes.

Fiber is an important part of the Body Shaping Diet because fiber fights fat and helps to maintain hormone balance.

TOO MUCH FIBER?

Some people experience discomfort when they switch to a high-fiber diet. Try to persevere because symptoms should lessen after a few days.

Symptoms can include increased flatulence, bloating, cramps, nausea and diarrhoea. This is often a result of the addition of wheat bran which can be an irritant to the intestine. I suggest you do not use this product.

The Body Shaping Diet is not for weight loss alone—more importantly the emphasis is on good health. We are encouraging foods which are soothing and protective to the digestive tract.

> **The reduction of meat products and the addition of foods rich in mucilage and vitamin A (rolled oats, yoghurt, yellow fruits and vegetables), will heal an inflamed colon, not irritate it.**

* If you have diverticulitis then you should avoid wholegrain products, little nuts, muesli and seeds as they can become trapped or caught in the bowel pockets. You should, however, still have fiber in your diet. You can grind seeds and nuts in a coffee grinder to make a fine powder which will not irritate those with diverticulitis.

MINIMISE FATS AND OILS

There is no doubt that excess fats and oils in your diet will stop you losing weight and will contribute to obesity. Where do you think the word 'fattening' originated?

Dietary fat that is not burned as energy is immediately stored as fat in your body.

Fats and oils are extremely high in calories and excess amounts will slow down your metabolic rate. They are difficult to digest and, if eaten in excess, may interfere with your ability to absorb nutrients from other foods.

Is it so surprising that you feel so sluggish and uncomfortable after eating foods with a high-fat content?

Many fats can be reduced in your diet simply by changing habits and cooking techniques.

A quick way to lessen the amount of fats in your diet is to stop buying processed foods. You know that packaged biscuits, cakes, pastry and fried foods are full of fat.

Reducing fats in your diet will also reduce your risk of heart disease and cancer.

Start making healthy choices and feel the benefit.

TYPES OF FATS

SATURATED FATS

The best way to identify a saturated fat is that it is solid at room temperature.

If you have a diet which is high in these fats you are more likely to have obesity, clogged arteries and you increase your risk of cancer of the breast, colon, ovaries and uterus.

Examples are fat in beef, pork, lamb, poultry, full-cream milk, cream, cheese, icecream, chocolate, ghee, butter, copha, dripping, suet, lard, coconut and palm oils.

UNSATURATED FATS

These are liquid or soft at room temperature.

Examples are fish oils, soft margarines, olive, linseed, canola, grapeseed, peanut, corn, safflower, sesame, soybean and sunflower oils.

These oils are a combination of mono-unsaturated and polyunsaturated oils.

The best choices of these oils are olive, canola or linseed.

Research shows that small quantities of these oils can be beneficial to the health of our arteries.

High-fat diets containing polyunsaturated oils and saturated fats have been shown to increase cancer growth in laboratory animals. So too have low-fat diets containing polyunsaturated oils.

There is no evidence at this time, of any links between mono-unsaturated oils and cancer growth.

None of these fats and oils are healthy if we subject them to heat processing or if we fry food in them!

MARGARINE OR BUTTER?

There is a great deal of debate and confusion regarding the use of butter or margarine.

Butter is a saturated fat and as such should be avoided if you are trying to achieve weight loss and/or reduce cholesterol levels.

The LYMPHATIC, GYNAEOID AND ANDROID body types must avoid butter completely and only use cold pressed vegetable or seed oils.

The THYROID body type will metabolize cholesterol foods better than the other body types and may include butter if they wish.

Margarine is a man-made product and many brands contain excessive chemicals to make them look and taste like butter. When analysed, this doesn't sound terribly healthy for us at all.

I suggest you try to avoid butter and margarine when following the weight loss programme—**STEP ONE**. Your body will be provided with enough 'healthy oils' from your daily allowance of nuts, seeds, grains and vegetable oils.

The addition of butter or margarine in your diet can quickly add unwanted calories.

1 level teaspoon of butter	=	36 cal/151 kJ
1 level teaspoon margarine	=	36 cal/151 kJ
1 level teaspoon low-fat margarine	=	18 cal/75 kJ

Try to eat sandwiches with a spreading like tahini, avocado and hummus instead of margarine and butter.

LINSEED OIL—A WISE CHOICE

Linseeds, like evening primrose oil, provide your body with some healthy omega 6 and omega 3 essential fatty acids and fiber. The following mixture can be made at home or purchased from a health food outlet.

**LSA = LINSEEDS (3 PARTS)
SUNFLOWER SEEDS (2 PARTS)
ALMONDS (1 PART)**

MIX AND GRIND TOGETHER INTO A FINE POWDER.

LSA is an excellent source of protein and contains calcium, phosphorus, potassium, iron, magnesium, copper, manganese, selenium, vitamin E, B group vitamins and vitamin A.

The linseed also has a laxative effect and this combination is an excellent addition to breakfast cereal, blended fruit shakes and can be added into many recipes to increase their nutritional value. Linseed is also know as flaxseed.

This mixture should always be purchased fresh (if already made at health food store), and stored in your refrigerator.

1 tablespoon LSA = 65 cal/273 kJ.

CHOLESTEROL

Cholesterol is a pearly, fatlike substance that is produced in your liver. It cannot dissolve in water or blood and it is transported in your body by lipoproteins. If your dietary cholesterol is high it may end up being deposited on the walls of your arteries. High-density lipoproteins are scavengers and help to clean up this cholesterol and carry it back to your liver to be reused.

You can't eat these lipoproteins because they are not found in foods. However you may increase the level of high-density lipoproteins by exercising, eating wisely, maintaining a healthy weight and not smoking.

Your body can produce all the cholesterol you need for health purposes without the need for added dietary cholesterol.

By having low-dietary cholesterol, your need for high-density lipoproteins is also low.

Generally it is ideal to have a blood cholesterol level of less than 200 mg/100 ml. Between 200 and 239 mg/100 ml is considered borderline high and over 240 mg/100 ml is considered to be a risk factor for cardio-vascular disease. So I encourage you to keep your cholesterol levels less than the 200 level.

Obesity also increases the risk of heart disease so a restriction in dietary fat is necessary on both counts.

While following the Body Shaping Diet you will benefit from a regime that is low in unhealthy fats and oils.

Reducing dietary saturated fat is only **one** of the methods of reducing cholesterol levels. Foods rich in saturated fats are all land animal products including full-cream dairy foods, shellfish, coconut milk and palm oil.

You must also **increase foods** which will help to lower cholesterol. They include **vitamin C rich foods, garlic, onion and foods containing soluble fiber** (see page 206).

Read labels on packaged food carefully for fat content.

SALT—SODIUM CHLORIDE

Salt is a compound of two elements, sodium and chloride. Forty per cent of salt is sodium and this is the mineral that we will discuss in this chapter.

Let's start by outlining that sodium deficiency is extremely rare, due to the fact that significant amounts of sodium are found in all foods except fruit.

Our nutritional requirement for sodium is only about 250–350 mg each day. If one level teaspoon of salt contains 2000 mg of sodium then it is easy to see why so many Americans eat too much salt.

It is not so surprising when you consider how much salt is added to processed and convenience foods, or what standard additions to the dinner table are the salt and pepper shakers.

Your tastebuds become accustomed to the flavour of salt. In fact, eating large amounts of salt can damage your tastebuds and you may not be experiencing the true flavors of your food.

There are several things that you need to do in order to reduce your sodium level. Read labels on food and avoid those products that contain salt or sodium in any form. Watch for hidden sodium in the form of flavour enhancers and preservatives like monosodium glutamate or MSG. Occasionally it is included in salt shakers at fast food outlets and adds a slightly different flavour to chips and chicken. Artificial sweeteners can also contain high levels of sodium.

Reducing your intake of processed and fast foods usually leads to a large reduction of dietary sodium levels.

Stop adding salt to your cooking and put away the salt shaker. At first you will miss the salty taste. In fact you may have strong cravings for several weeks but they will pass. If you can persevere, after a couple of months your tastebuds will come to life and you will be able to taste the true flavors of food once again.

> People with high blood pressure or fluid retention are usually advised by their health practitioner to reduce their salt intake. This is because research has shown a strong connection between these disorders and high dietary sodium levels.

The Body Shaping Diet allows you to add roasted nuts, seeds, herbs, tasty sauces and low-calorie dressings to your food. If you are a salt user, the addition of these flavorings will help you to overcome the need to add salt.

TEA AND COFFEE

The Body Shaping Diet allows you up to four cups of tea or coffee daily.

If you can only drink tea or coffee with sugar, it might be wiser to avoid it unless you can become used to drinking it without. Or you may prefer herbal tea, which can be taken more freely and is easier to drink without sweeteners.

For tea drinkers I recommend that you limit tannin-containing tea to two cups per day. Tannin is a strong astringent and it can reduce your body's ability to absorb iron, which can lead to anemia.

Two brands of tannin-free tea that come to mind are Celestial Seasonings and Lipton Soothing moments tea. They are readily available at the supermarket or health food store and even hardened tea drinkers will be delighted with their flavor.

Coffee is a stimulant that contains high levels of caffeine. If you enjoy a cup of coffee and have no bad effects from it, then 2–4 cups a day will not be harmful to you.

Sensitivity to caffeine can bring on palpitations, anxiety attacks and migraine headaches. It can raise blood pressure, interfere with healthy sleeping patterns and weaken the muscle tone of your bladder. If you have any of these problems you should avoid coffee and other foods that contain caffeine such as cola drinks, chocolate and tea.

Women with lumpy, sore breasts will benefit by removing caffeine from their diet.

The alternatives are dandelion or cereal beverages, which contain no caffeine and are excellent coffee alternatives.

Do not include tea or coffee when you calculate your daily water consumption.

ALCOHOL

Alcohol is hideously fattening so it can be extremely difficult to achieve weight loss, maintain good health and include alcohol in your regime all at the same time. Alcohol is very high in calories compared to other sources of energy. It yields 7 cal/29 kJ per gram compared to protein or carbohydrate foods which yield 4 cal/17 kJ per gram.

For women, one or two alcoholic drinks a day should not pose any serious health problems, however you must reduce alcohol in order to lose body fat.

Remember that alcohol is a depressant which slows down the speed at which you digest food. It is also destructive to nutrients and can reduce your calcium levels, paving the way for osteoporosis.

Even though it may be part of your social habits, I encourage you to say no. A couple of drinks may weaken your resolve and you are more likely to eat the wrong foods or, more seriously, substitute alcohol for food.

Once you reach **STEP TWO**—Maintenance, you may introduce one or two alcoholic drinks a day if you wish, although we do not recommend this. One or two drinks on the weekend is safe.

For now, eliminate alcohol and know that you are not adding empty calories. Instead, replace it with water, mineral water or soda water with a twist of lime or lemon, or a fresh fruit or vegetable juice.

ABDOMINAL SWELLING AND DIGESTIVE DISCOMFORT

Many women complain of fullness or bloating after eating. There is often an increase in wind or flatulence and occasionally pain or burning. This may be caused by physical problems such as hiatus hernia, enzyme insufficiency or inflammatory disorders such as colitis, diverticulitis or ulceration. Other causes may be candida, stress, food intolerance and sometimes poor food combinations.

Listed below are some self-help ideas for some of these problems.

HIATUS HERNIA. Eat smaller meals. Do not fill your stomach with large quantities of food or liquids as this causes the stomach to 'balloon' out and leads to discomfort and pain. Avoid beer and carbonated drinks. Do not drink with meals.

INFLAMMATORY DISORDERS. Do not allow yourself to have long periods without any food. Save your fruit servings for in between meals.

Select foods which are rich in vitamin A, such as yellow fruits and vegetables, to heal and soothe the tissues. Eat foods which will soothe and protect the digestive tract such as rolled oats, yoghurt, pawpaw, pumpkin, sweet potato and rice.

Do not drink tea, coffee or alcoholic beverages. Coloneze powder and FiberTone powder are excellent for irritable bowel syndrome and inflammatory bowel disorders.

Try one or two small glasses of raw cabbage juice daily.

WIND OR FLATULENCE. Do not rush meals and maintain good posture whilst eating. Try eliminating all fermented foods such as vinegars, chutneys, soy sauce etc. Remove all sugar and foods containing added sugar from your diet. Reduce your intake of yeast by eating yeast-free bread and eliminating alcohol.

Try eating your fruit before your meal rather than after, and do not eat fruit with bread, such as banana or apple sandwiches. Some people find that combinations of tomato and bread, or meat and bread can also lead to discomfort.

You may find that taking a supplement of Digestive Enzymes may help. These do not stop you producing enzymes, they simply provide you with extra enzymes to assist digestive processes.

Herbal teas which would help are chamomile, peppermint, ginger, aniseed, caraway, cinnamon, cloves, lemon balm and dill.

CHAPTER EIGHT

CELLULITE

Cellulite is the word used to describe the lumpy uneven type of fat that accumulates on the buttocks and limbs of many women. It is rather unsightly because it gives the tissues underlying the skin (subcutaneous tissues) an 'orange peel' or 'cottage cheese' look.

Cellulite has been studied by doctors for many years and it has been categorised by several medical names such as lipodystrophy, mesenchymal disease or liposclerosis.

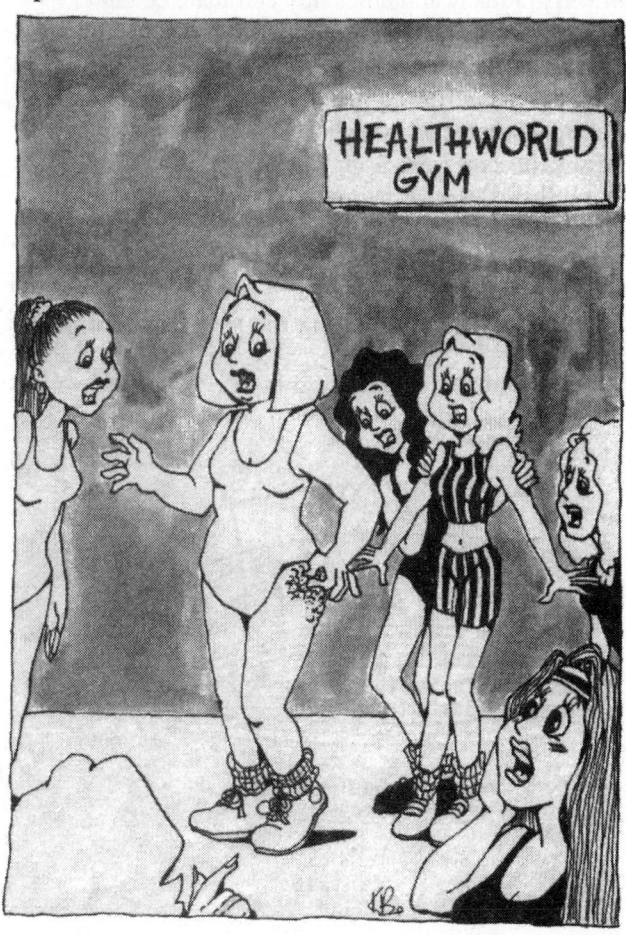

If we compare cellulite fat to normal fat we find that in the former there are abnormal, physical and chemical changes.

In women with cellulite, pinching of the skin produces a 'mattress appearance' with bulging and pitting of the fatty layer. On deep palpation of this layer one may be able to feel tender nodules of fat trapped inside hardened connective tissue.

There are several causes of cellulite:

hereditary factors   **lymphatic factors**
intestinal factors   **hormonal factors**
circulatory factors   **lifestyle factors**

The Body Shaping Diet and exercise programme takes all these factors into account and will gradually and efficiently eliminate cellulite.

Cellulite is most common in the gynaeoid-shaped woman where it accumulates on the thighs and buttocks. In the lymphatic-shaped woman it accumulates on the legs, upper arms, buttocks and abdomen and is worsened by poor drainage of fluid through the swollen lymphatic vessels. If any of the four body shapes become overweight, cellulite may develop as metabolism of the fatty tissues becomes increasingly underactive.

Diagram 9 shows us what fat tissue looks like under the microscope. If cellulite develops in fat tissue, it looks abnormal under the microscope and the fat cell chambers become swollen and pinched by the connective tissue bands seen in our diagram. This results in a restriction of the blood circulation through the tiny capillaries supplying the fat cells, which in turn reduces

Diagram 9

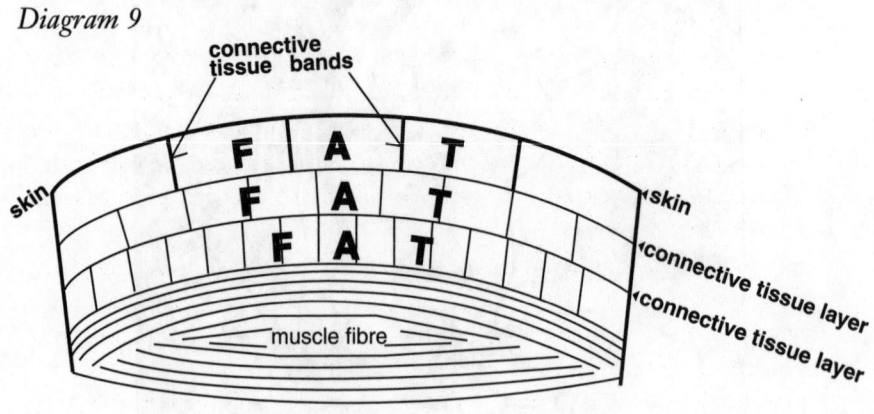

Anatomy of Fat Tissue
(note 3 layers of fat)

oxygen supply to the fat cells thus reducing their metabolism. This is why cellulite is so hard to lose. The connective tissue layers and bands become tougher and less elastic, trapping fluids and waste products between them and pinching the tiny ends of nerve fibres, which may cause areas affected by cellulite to ache. Eventually, in well-developed cellulite we see stagnation and hardening of all structures in the fat layers, so that the tissue takes on a lifeless quality—a bit like hard lumpy cheese.

To lose this cellulite the areas of fat affected must be revitalized and transformed bringing back active metabolic processes within each fat cell. To achieve complete success we must have a plan of attack containing several strategies.

Firstly the Body Shaping Diet should be followed for your particular body shape.

There are also some general strategies that must be applied for all body shapes afflicted with cellulite—that is if they want to lose all their cellulite.

GENERAL STRATEGIES

Avoid saturated fats from fried foods, processed foods, all dairy products, fatty meats such as pork, organ meats, lamb, battery chickens, creamy or rich sauces and gravies, cakes and biscuits made with butter or processed fats.

Some women will find that their cellulite will not disappear completely while they continue to consume saturated fats. I remember one young woman with cellulite on her upper outer thighs that refused to budge while she continued with a diet containing three serves of low-fat dairy products daily. Only after eliminating all dairy products and red meats was she able to shed her cellulite.

If this is your case, then it is quite safe to completely eliminate all dairy products and red meats until your cellulite disappears. You are what you eat— if you are eating saturated fats and not metabolising them, then they will be laid down as fat and perhaps cellulite in your body. Thus, for a limited time, until the cellulite disappears, you may need a diet free of all dairy products, red meat, and poultry.

While on such a diet, I advise a supplement of calcium 800 mg daily, organic iron 100 mg daily and vitamin B12 50 mcg daily. If you stick to a dairy and meat free diet for more than three months, please see your doctor to check your levels of vitamin B12 and iron.

For those wishing to lose cellulite quickly, the red meat, poultry and dairy free diet is superb. To make sure you do not become deficient in protein (in amino acids) I advise that you get first-class protein daily either from fish or by combining grains, nuts, seeds and legumes for at least one meal every day.

Avoid processed foods containing colorings, preservatives and flavorings, such as fizzy drinks, boxed and packaged cereals and meals, cakes and biscuits found in most supermarkets, foods made from white flour and sugar and foods high in salt.

Avoid alcohol—restrict your alcohol to one or two glasses on the weekend, or if you are not fussed, avoid it completely.

Avoid snacks between meals—restrict these to raw celery, carrots or apples only and eat only three meals a day. Diabetics will need modification of this under supervision from their specialist.

Detoxify the body—the fat cells in cellulite are literally choked and 'suffocated' by stagnant fluids and waste products trapped in hardened connective tissues. To transform these half-dead fat cells, we must first detoxify them or give them a 'spring cleaning'. This can be done by increasing your consumption of **raw** or living foods—such as sprouted seeds, **raw** fruits and vegetables. Some women prefer to do this by eating only raw fruits and vegetables for one or two days of every week—a type of 'raw food fasting' if you like.

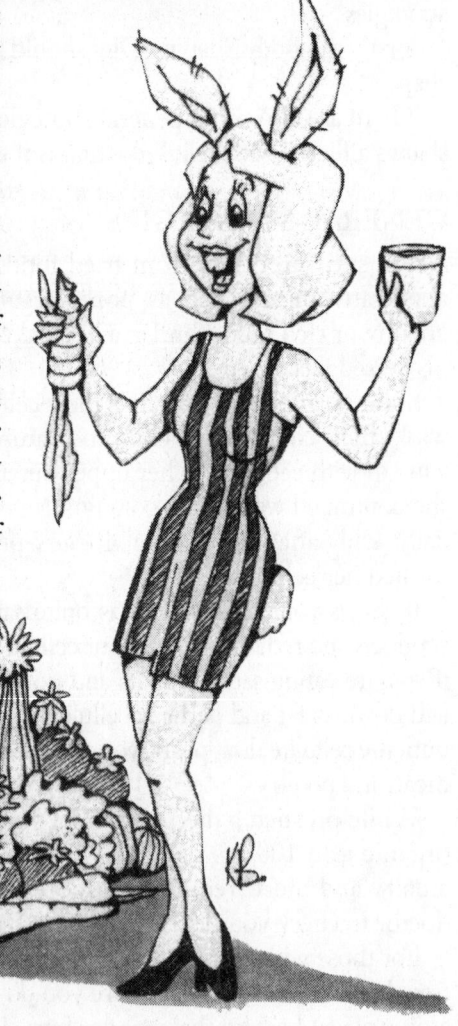

Alternatively, you may elect to have a fruit-only breakfast, which is a great way to cleanse the liver and bowels for the start of the day.

I am often amazed by the number of women who rarely eat salads of raw vegetables except on hot summer days, as they see this as 'Bugs Bunny food' and not the foundation of a healthy diet. Our mothers and grand-mothers often inculcated this misconception during our childhood.

My recommendation, not only for cellulite sufferers but for all women desirous of good health and a longer life span, is to eat one **huge raw salad**—full of fresh raw vegetables of all varieties—**every day.** Dressings can be made with lemon, lime or apple cider vinegar and a touch of cold pressed olive oil, sunflower, safflower or grapeseed oil. You may put avo-cado in your salads as it is free of cholesterol; three avocados per week being the maximum.

To flavor the salads use fresh aromatic herbs and vegetables such as parsley, mint, coriander, basil, thyme, chives and/or finely chopped spring onions. A rather exotic taste to the salad can be obtained by using fresh ginger passed through a garlic press. For those who like more bite, use a dash of chilli or soy sauce, garlic or black pepper.

The battle of cellulite will never be won unless you become a lover of raw foods every day. Make sure you chew slowly and thoroughly!

Another vital tool to detoxify and revitalize fatty tissues is to drink pure water—one and a half to two quarts daily is the target. This must be taken as water only or unsweetened herbal teas and not in the form of ordinary tea and coffee.

EXERCISES FOR CELLULITE

Exercise used as part of a programme to reduce cellulite and help to keep it off needs to be **isotonic.** This means it needs to take you through a broad range of large movements such as in cycling, swimming, running, power walking or rowing. This kind of exercise shortens and lengthens your muscles rhythmically.

You need to become fit all over, that is why aerobic exercise, especially the low-impact type, is extremely beneficial for cellulite. The fitter you are the lower your resting heart rate is, which means you can deal better with stress without such a large build-up of chemical by-products in your system.

The best exercise is definitely a constant low intensity, rhythmical type where you are using the large muscle groups at an intensity that increases your heart rate to 60 per cent of your maximum heart rate. This is called your tar-get heart rate and it is necessary to achieve this if you want to increase your metabolic rate and so increase the rate at which you burn up excess fat.

To find your **maximum heart rate**, subtract your age from 220.

To find your **target heart rate**, multiply the above figure (220 minus your age) by 0.6.

For example, if you are 40 years old your maximum heart rate = 220 minus 40 = 180 beats per minute. Your target heart rate = 180 x 0.6 = 108 beats per minute. By reaching your target heart rate via exercise you will increase your metabolic rate.

To reduce cellulite you should leave no longer than forty-eight hours between each session of exercise and you can work out for anything between fifteen to sixty minutes a session, three to five times a week. Ideally, you could do five, thirty-minute sessions as that would keep your metabolic rate up and running, therefore preventing the build up of cellulite.

Massage and hydrotherapy are also excellent in helping to stimulate lymphatic drainage and reduce cellulite. Massage with an anti-cellulite preparation and anti-cellulite gloves or a mitt for massage can be very useful and should be done two to three times per week.

EXERCISE

This is an essential part of your weight-loss and body shaping programme. Exercise will improve the health of your heart and lungs, regulate your desire for food and speed up your weight loss. Regular exercise greatly improves our moods because it stimulates the brain's production of endorphin chemicals which are natural anti-depressants. Your exercise routine should be done every day and if it is difficult to get out of the house, you can do your exercise at home while listening to stimulating music. If you fall into the very over-weight range, the best exercise to start with is gentle swimming or walking. As you lose weight, more strenuous exercises such as aerobics or jogging can be started.

Be on the look-out for opportunities to exercise, such as getting off the bus a few stops earlier, taking the stairs instead of the elevator, leaving your car at home or stopping for a walk in the park at lunch or tea breaks. Some days you may feel like putting it off, but try to force yourself to overcome laziness and lethargy because the results are many times worth the effort. The more you exercise the better you will look and feel. If you burn up 250 calories (1050 kJ) daily with exercise, this would result in a weekly weight loss of half a pound. If you burn up 500 calories (2100 kJ) daily with exercise, this would result in a weekly weight loss of just over a pound.

ACTIVITY	CALORIES BURNED PER MINUTE
VERY LIGHT e.g. dusting slow walking, yoga	2 (8.4 kJ)
MODERATE e.g. brisk walking energetic gardening scrubbing the floor	3.5-7 (14.7-29.4 kJ)
HEAVY e.g. running, aerobics swimming laps, rowing weight running	>7.5 (>31.5 kJ)

BODY SHAPING EXERCISE PROGRAMME

The Body Shaping Diet will allow you to lose weight from where you want to but we also encourage you to do a daily programme of exercises designed to:

1. Warm you up.
2. Stretch and relax the muscles and joints.
3. Firm and tone the muscles so that your new shape will look firm and contoured.

By doing our simple and balanced programme of exercises you will be able to achieve your new body shape more quickly. Our exercises can be done in 20–30 minutes and should be done every day.

The exercises are designed for women who don't have a regular exercise programme and you don't need to be fit to begin! If you have any medical problems it is wise to check with your doctor before you begin any exercise programme. For those with any joint or back problems, consult a physiotherapist who can modify these exercises specifically for you to avoid any injury or sprains. We also encourage you to do regular (2–3 times per week) recreational or aerobic exercise to promote overall cardiovascular and muscular fitness. Such exercises may include brisk walking, jogging, aerobics or sports such as rowing, tennis, basketball, scuba diving or golf. Tai chi or yoga can be very relaxing and improve muscular co-ordination, balance and posture. Aqua-aerobics or swimming are excellent exercises for all women but especially for those with joint or back pain. Many a chronic back ache has been cured with regular swimming alone.

One final word of warning—you should never force yourself to do or persist with any exercise which causes pain or discomfort.

WARM-UP

Take a brisk walk for at least 15 minutes daily making sure that you relax the shoulders and swing your arms freely. Keep your body tall and straight and stretch the legs by taking large strides, generally this will cause the pulse rate to rise to between 90 and 120 beats per minute. Count your pulse at the wrist for 10 seconds and multiply this number by 6 to give your pulse rate per minute. If you are a lymphatic type, walking is particularly beneficial in reducing swelling and puffiness of the legs and you should try to do 30 minutes of brisk walking daily.

Warm-up

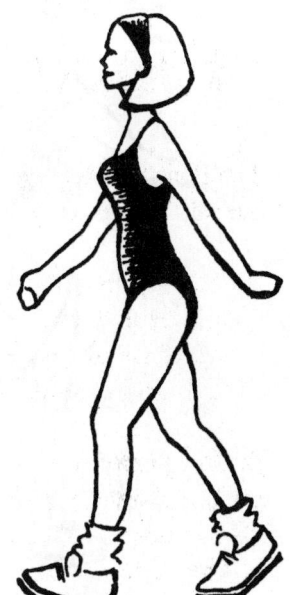

STRETCHING—*for five minutes*
Stretching the muscles and joint ligaments in a gentle and gradual way will make you flexible and reduce sprains and injury. All exercises to be repeated on each side.

1. Place one arm horizontally in front of your upper chest, flex it at the elbow and pull from the elbow to stretch the back of your arm and shoulder. Hold for 10 seconds.

1. 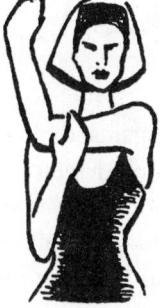 2. 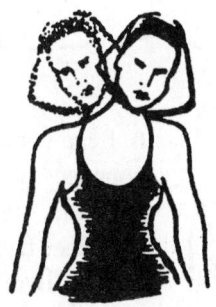 3.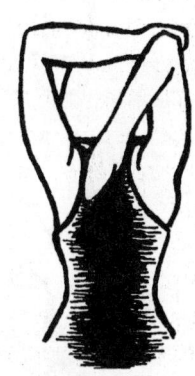

Stretching

2. Move your neck slowly to the right and then to the left—hold each side for 10 seconds.

3. Raise your arm behind your head and bend and stretch gently until the hand reaches the middle of your upper back—hold for 10 seconds.

4.

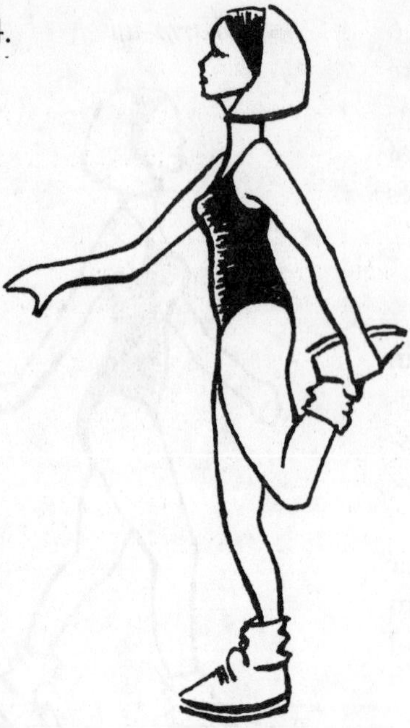

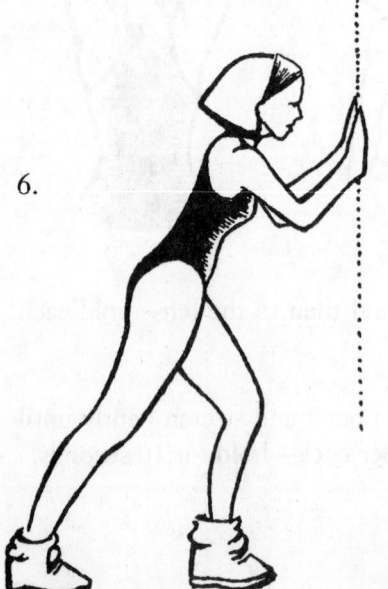

4. Hold your foot against the corresponding buttock (bottom) to stretch the front of the thigh (quadriceps muscle)—hold for 10 seconds.

5. Lying with your back on the floor or on a rug, pull your leg toward your chest. It is important to keep your lower back flat and your head on the floor—hold this stretch for 10 seconds.

Stretching

5.

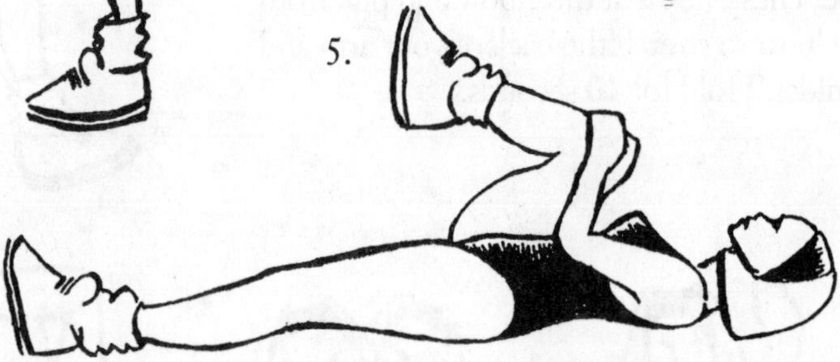

6.

6. Lean your hands against the wall with your feet approximately 1 metre (3 feet) from the wall. Lean into the wall keeping your feet flat and feel your calf muscles stretch. Bend one knee forward toward the wall keeping your back leg straight with its foot flat and toes pointed straight ahead. Press your heels to the floor and hold for 10 seconds.

Exercises to Strengthen, Tone and Firm the Muscles

BOTTOM EXERCISES

1. Lie on your back with your knees bent and feet flat on the ground. Lift your bottom from the floor keeping your back straight. Do one set of 5 with feet apart, and one set of 5 with feet together.

This exercise will firm and tone the muscles of the bottom and front thighs and is ideal for gynaeoid-shaped women. If you want to increase its effectiveness do four sets of 5 (both feet apart and together) every day.

2. Get on your forearms and knees and keeping your back straight, stretch one leg backwards, parallel to the floor flexing your foot. Bring the knee forward under your stomach and then push the leg backwards while holding in your stomach muscles. While the leg is back, bend it a little at the knee and lift it slightly (just 2 inches) skyward, keeping your foot flexed. Do 10 on each side.

This exercise firms the muscles of the bottom and back of the thighs (hamstrings) and is vital for women who want to reduce the size and floppiness of the back of their bottom. Gynaeoid-shaped women should try to do 20 to 30 of these on each side.

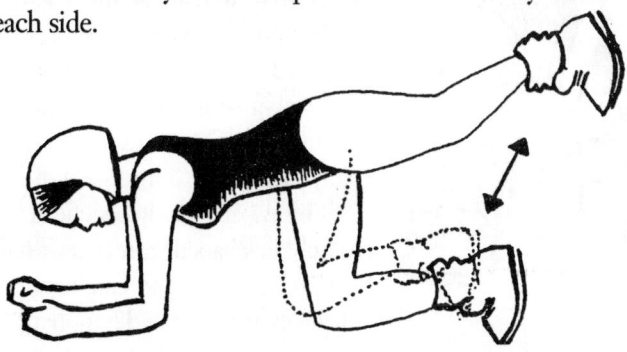

ABDOMINAL EXERCISES

These are excellent for all body types but especially for android-shaped women who tend towards fat excess on the upper and lower abdomen (known disparagingly as a pot belly).

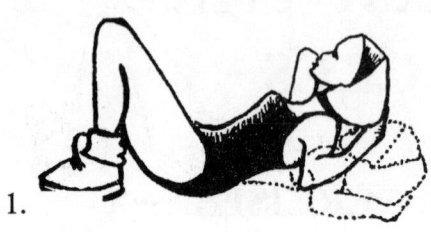

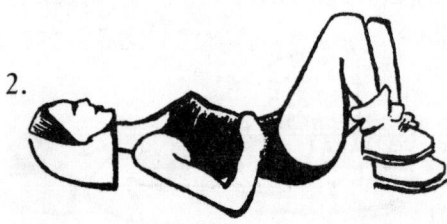

1. *Sit-ups* will firm and flatten the upper abdominal muscles. Lie on the floor, knees bent, with the soles of your feet flat on the floor and close to your bottom. Press your lower back into the floor and place your hands behind your head with elbows out behind you. Lift your shoulders and head off the ground a few inches. Start with one set of 10 and gradually build up to three sets of 10 each day. If tired, make sure you rest before each set. Exhale while lifting.

2. To firm and tone the lower abdominal muscles lie on your back on a firm surface. Bend your knees and place your feet flat on the ground and your fingers next to your umbilicus. Raise one leg upwards bringing your foot about 3 inches off the ground. Then lift up your other leg and hold both feet up for 5–10 seconds, then relax both feet back on the ground. Start with 10 of these and gradually build to three sets of 10 each day.

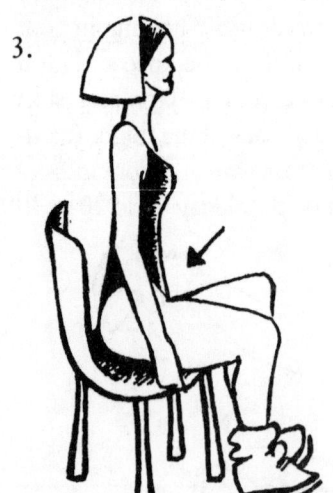

3. *To firm and shape the waist.* Sit on a stool and gradually tighten the stomach muscles until they feel tight and firm. Hold them tight for 5–10 seconds and then relax them while breathing out fully. Do this exercise 10 times and gradually increase it to three sets of 10 per day.

This is particularly beneficial for android and lymphatic-shaped women as it reduces a protuberant abdomen and encourages decongestion of the pelvic veins and lymphatic vessels.

LEG EXERCISES

1. *Inner thigh.* Lie on a firm surface and push your back into the ground. Bend your knees and place the soles of your feet together, still keeping your feet on the ground. Now squeeze your knees together and hold for 5–10 seconds. If this causes any discomfort on the knees, place a small folded towel between the knee joints to avoid pressure while squeezing them together. Start with one set of 5 working up to four sets of 5.

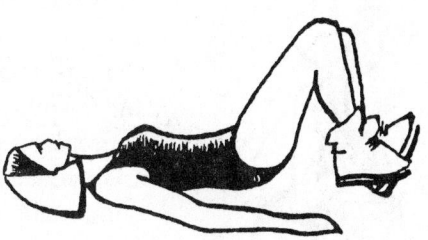

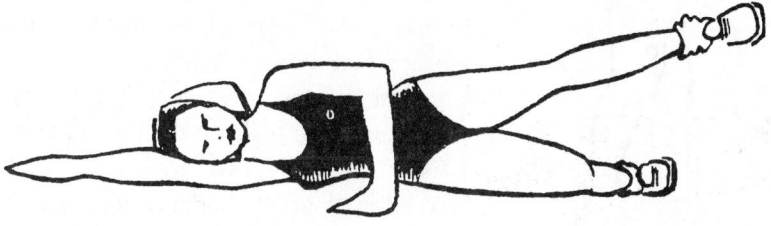

2. *Outer thigh.* Lie on your side on a firm surface with your upper leg straight and your lower leg bent at a 90° angle. Lift your upper leg straight up as high as possible, then slowly lower it down. Keep your hips one above the other (i.e. don't lean forward or backward) and your toes pointing forward. Repeat lifting and lowering your upper leg 10 times, then roll over to the other side and repeat.

This exercise firms and tones the muscles of the buttocks and outer thigh and is great for gynaeoid-shaped women wanting to reduce their bottoms and outer thighs.

ARMS AND CHEST

After losing weight many women find that the muscles of the back and the upper arm (triceps) remain loose and floppy. This can be avoided with these exercises.

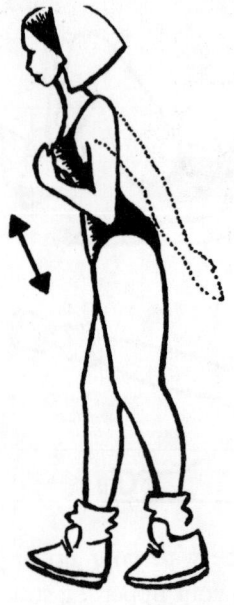

1. Stand with one foot in front of the other placing your body weight slightly forwards. Bend your elbows, pressing them into the sides of your abdomen. Push each arm backwards in a squeezing motion. Do one set of 10 and build up to three sets of 10 for each arm. You may find it comfortable to stand alongside a cupboard and balance your body weight on the top of the cupboard with the non-exercising hand. This exercise can also be done using small hand-held weights of half to one pound.

This exercise is great for thyroid-shaped women wanting to build up their upper arms.

2. Sit on a stool, bring your arms up to shoulder height and bend the elbows. Slowly move the arms forward until the elbows and wrists touch in front of your chest and face, then move them

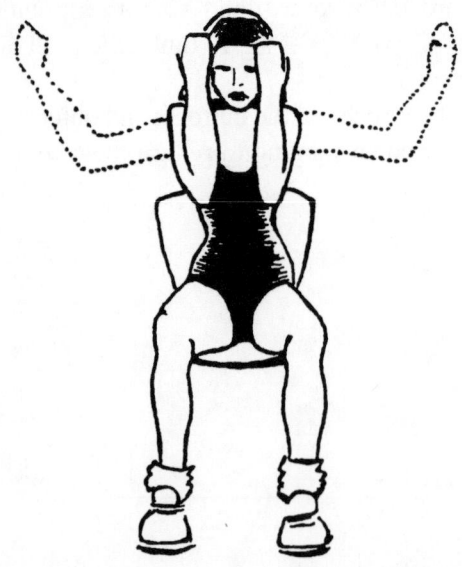

back to the side keeping them at shoulder height. Squeeze the arm muscles as you go. Start with 10 of these and gradually increase to three sets of 10.

3. *Push-ups*. Begin on your hands and knees, with hands parallel to each other and a little more than shoulder width apart. The wider apart your hands are, the harder you will work your chest muscles. Lower your body down, keeping it straight, until your chest only touches the floor, then push yourself straight up to the starting position. Repeat 5 times and gradually build up to 10 to 20 push-ups each day.

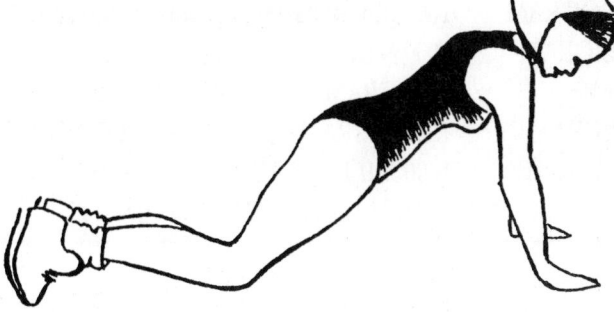

TABLE OF CONVERSIONS AND SYMBOLS

CAL	CALORIE	1 CALORIE	= 4.2 KILOJOULES
kJ	KILOJOULE	4.2 KILOJOULES	= 1 CALORIE
mcg	MICROGRAM	1000 MICROGRAMS	= 1 MILLIGRAM
mg	MILLIGRAM	1000 MILLIGRAMS	= 1 GRAM
g	GRAM	1000 GRAMS	= 1 KILOGRAM
kg	KILOGRAM	1 KILOGRAM	= 2.2 POUNDS
ml	MILLILITRE	1000 MILLILITRES	= 1 LITRE
		500 MILLILITRES	= 1 PINT

CHAPTER NINE

EATING DISORDERS

BULIMIA

Sarah was eighteen when she first discovered that making herself vomit was a way of controlling her weight. It was partly accidental—after a large meal she felt bloated and making herself vomit afterwards seemed easy. It was the start, however, of a pattern of making herself vomit more and more often. She felt bad about doing it, hated being physically sick and began to avoid eating so she would not 'have to' be sick. This meant that when she did eat she felt overly full very quickly and had an intense urge to vomit. She was vomiting three or four times every day by the time she decided she needed help to stop. She had difficulty coping with work and her part-time study because all her energy was used in thinking about eating and controlling her weight. She felt ashamed about her eating and vomiting and hated having to lie about it to keep it secret.

Sarah was suffering from bulimia, which today has become quite a common disorder in Western societies. Many of the features of bulimia overlap with those of anorexia but bulimic individuals tend to maintain their normal weight. When diagnosing bulimia doctors and psychologists have a technical definition which includes: a sense of lack of control, making your-self vomit, using laxatives or fluid tablets and strict dieting or exercising in order to prevent weight gain. People with bulimia also generally have an over-concern with body weight and shape, similar to that seen in anorexia.

Apart from being unpleasant and distasteful, making yourself vomit is not an effective strategy for losing weight. Because it disrupts the body's natural way of obtaining nutrients from food, most people with bulimia develop other symptoms such as poor concentration, depression, moodiness, irritability and fatigue.

Repeated vomiting or purging can also be dangerous. The major medical risks come from changes in the body's natural salt balance, which commonly causes tiredness and muscle weakness but can also cause the heart to beat irregularly, or even stop. Acid from the stomach also erodes tooth enamel and causes tooth decay.

Today there are many forms of treatment available. All involve learning something about the disorder and most involve coming to some understanding of the meaning of the illness for the individual.

Once the disorder is established it can be very difficult to stop by yourself and professional advice is generally the most reliable way of getting better.

Different therapists have different approaches and most will tailor the type of therapy to the needs and personality of the individual. It is important, firstly, to learn something about bulimia and about healthy patterns of eating and nutrition. A dietitian with experience in treating bulimia can be a great help with this. The most common psychological treatments involve a form of behaviour therapy called cognitive behaviour therapy. There are many elements to this but the focus of the treatment is on modifying the irrational thoughts that are associated with the binge eating and vomiting.

Many patients need to deal with painful feelings coming from parts of their life unrelated directly to food and other forms of psychotherapy may be most helpful for this. Bulimia is often exacerbated by life stress and learning other ways of dealing with this will generally be part of a treatment package. Your therapist will advise about the best treatment.

Some medications can be helpful for treating bulimia, particularly if depression is a major part of the problem.

Hospitalization in a specialised eating disorder unit is generally effective at breaking the bulimia cycle. Treatment in hospital is essentially similar to that outlined above but is more intensive. It often involves group programmes and allows eating behaviour to be changed in a more structured way with twenty-four hour support from experienced staff. Because in the long run the changes in behaviour need to occur in the person's natural environment, hospitalization is generally kept in reserve for people who are not able to solve the problem with outpatient treatment.

Some people are reluctant to seek professional help because of embarrassment or cost. They may be able to benefit from a self-help programme and for them a good resource could be a book called *Fighting with Food* by G. F. Huon and L. B. Brown, which is published by NSW University Press, Australia. This is available at most bookshops and libraries.

Without treatment, bulimia tends to continue over many years, often varying in severity in relation to stress. For some sufferers, the symptoms are quite incapacitating. A treatment programme will usually take several months. Response to treatment is generally good, enabling people to get on with their lives without pervasive concerns about weight, shape and food.

This section on bulimia was written by Doctor Greg McKeough, a consultant psychiatrist who works with women suffering with eating disorders.

ANOREXIA NERVOSA—THE HUNGER WITHIN

Anorexia nervosa is the medical term for self-induced starvation. 'Anorexia' means loss of appetite and the word 'nervosa' indicates its relationship to an imbalance in the nervous system. In Westernised societies, anorexia nervosa is not an uncommon disorder, it affects one in every two hundred women under the age of twenty-five and typically has its onset in adolescence or the twenties. The anorexic woman becomes fully pre-occupied with her body weight and shape and has a morbid fear of becoming fat. In many cases she would rather die than become fat! She pursues thinness relentlessly and fears food because she may not be able to control her weight if she eats one skerrick of food too much. Her rigid dieting is often accompanied by a rigorous schedule of arduous exercise that she forces herself to do in spite of her exhausted state. Eating may be followed by self-induced vomiting or ingestion of laxatives and purgative drugs. This can result in damaged teeth, swollen salivary glands and severe imbalances in body minerals.

I have called anorexia nervosa 'the hunger within' because sufferers are not only starving physically but also deep inside their emotional being there is a hunger. They are hungry for love, acceptance, admiration, independence, maturity, indeed for life. But they are in a paradox because although they want these things, they are too frightened to let themselves evolve and develop enough to grasp them. Fundamentally, the anorexic woman is terribly insecure, lacks confidence and has poor self-esteem, which makes it difficult for her to face the normal phases of life as she grows up. She may fear her sexuality and the prospects of sexual relationships, responsibility, childbirth or parenthood and tries to escape these things by starving herself into a childlike or pre-adolescent state. She wants to be a 'Peter Pan' never growing up and living in a fantasy world where she controls her life with a protective suit of armor in the form of childlike thinness. She regresses to a pre-adolescent physical state.

Her fear of womanhood and sexuality may be based on a poor relationship with her father, sexual abuse, incest or rejection from boyfriends or close friends.

Because adolescence brings the first prospects of independence and sexuality, it is not surprising that this is the most common time for anorexia nervosa to begin.

In general, the anorexic woman is resistant to help and does not go along to a doctor of her own volition to seek treatment for her weight loss. In the majority of cases she is brought along to a doctor by a family member or close friend who is concerned by her loss of appetite and weight. The anorexic woman usually makes light of her thinness and is evasive or untruthful in answering questions about her food intake. She will often state that she is still too fat and desires to lose more weight, even though to all others she appears painfully thin; this is due to her distorted self body image.

Physical Signs

A woman suffering with severe anorexia nervosa will at some stage of her illness have the following physical signs of her disease:

1. A body weight less than 80 per cent of the average body weight for her age and height and in many cases she may weigh much less. Her body mass index will generally be less than 15.
2. Loss of regular menstrual periods due to her low levels of estrogen.
3. Soft downy hair growing on her limbs and face.
4. A slow heart rate, low blood pressure and cold hands and feet. This is due to a general slowing down of her metabolic rate, which occurs as a protective mechanism to slow down the rate at which her body consumes or lives off its own tissues.
5. Loss and wasting of muscular tissues.
6. Vitamin and mineral deficiencies.

Treatment

The aim of therapy is to restore body weight into the normal range. To do this it is necessary to supervise the food intake and in severe cases this is best done in hospital. There are hospitals that have special programmes and inpatient eating disorder units. Women with severe anorexia nervosa will usually spend eight to twelve weeks in hospital.

Strategies that are helpful are individual counselling (psychotherapy), group therapy, nutritional counselling, body shape examinations, as well as analysis of eating behaviour.

In severe cases forced feeding in hospital to save a life may be required. One can never be complacent or treat anorexia as a minor illness. It is a serious emotional and physical disorder that carries a significant risk of death.

Forced feeding will not provide a long-term solution and indeed patience and persistence are required because to overcome anorexia nervosa years of psychotherapy are often necessary.

During psychotherapy it is useful to explore childhood patterns of eating as there may have been a power struggle between the child and parents using food as the weapon. Other issues such as body image, self esteem, expectations, assertiveness and sexuality need to be explored. Techniques of behaviour modification, self hypnosis, meditation and relaxation are useful to increase self confidence and soften the high and often rigid standards that anorexic women impose upon themselves. Anorexic women may be obsessive perfectionists and they need to learn how to be kinder and gentler on themselves.

If the anorexia is associated with mental illness such as severe depression, psychosis or schizophrenia, anti-depressant or tranquillizing drugs are required before other measures can be started.

The biggest hurdle to overcome is the resistance of the anorexic woman to fully partake of the treatment programme and that is why one in every ten anorexic women continue to be thin and unwell.

Women with anorexia nervosa can only use the Body Shaping Diet under supervision from their doctor as they will need more calories than this to get their body mass index back into the normal range of 19 to 25.

Nutritional Supplements for Women with Eating Disorders

Women with anorexia nervosa and bulimia have abnormalities in the function of their immune and hormonal systems. There are often imbalances in the chemical processes inside the body cells with reduced energy production occurring.

Imbalances of this sort often cause fatigue, extreme mood changes, deep depressions, disturbed thoughts and cravings for refined sugars.

These symptoms can be greatly reduced by the regular daily ingestion of specific nutritional supplements.

Women with eating disorders need:

1. Niacin or Nicotinamide, 250 mg with each meal. This is also known as vitamin B3.
2. Essential fatty acids—with meals. Flaxseed oil capsules–2 capsules twice daily.
3. Vitamin B Complex, 1 daily with main meal.
4. Bone Joint and Cartilage Nutrient Powder – one teaspoon daily.
5. Iron amino acid chelate, 100 mg daily taken with vitamin C or citrus fruits.
6. Zinc chelate 30–50 mg daily.

The improvement that these nutritional supplements produce is truly remarkable and I cannot stress enough the importance of taking them regularly if you are a woman battling with an eating disorder.

GLOSSARY

ADRENAL GLANDS Two small glands situated on top of the kidneys, which secrete steroid hormones and the stress hormone adrenalin.

AMINO ACIDS The building blocks of the body's protein. Ten of the amino acids are essential dietary components as they cannot be synthesized by the body. Dietary protein can only be considered first class if it contains all the ten essential amino acids. First class protein can be obtained from animal and dairy products and also by combining any three of the following: nuts, grains, seeds, legumes at one meal.

ANABOLIC STEROIDS Male hormones which stimulate the growth of bone and muscle.

ANDROGEN Male hormone.

ANOREXIA Loss of appetite.

ANTI-MALE HORMONE A hormone which blocks the synthesis and effects of male hormones and is capable of reversing masculine body features.

ANTIOXIDANT Substances such as vitamins A, C and E, beta-carotene and selenium, which protect the cellular structures from oxidative damage caused by free radicals.

BIOFLAVONOIDS Bioflavonoids, sometimes referred to as vitamin P, are found in plants along with vitamin C and exert a beneficial effect upon the walls of the blood and lymphatic vessels. This is very helpful for women troubled with fluid retention and puffy limbs.

BODY MASS INDEX (BMI) The BMI is a scientific way of examining 'fatness' and 'thinness' and is worked out according to the formula BMI = weight (kilogram) / height squared (metres^2). The normal BMI for women ranges from 19 to 25 kg/m^2 and many hormonal and menstrual problems can be overcome by keeping weight in the normal BMI range.

BODY TYPE There are four body shapes or physiques, namely gynaeoid, thyroid, android and lymphatic.

BULIMIA A disorder of eating characterised by lack of control, making yourself vomit after eating, using laxatives, diuretics and strict dieting to prevent weight gain.

CAFFEINE A central nervous system stimulant found in tea, coffee and cola drinks.

CARDIOVASCULAR DISEASE Disease of the system of the blood

circulation comprising the heart and blood vessels.

CHOLESTEROL A constituent of all animal fats. It is found in the blood in two forms: 1. High Density Lipo-protein (HDL) which protects against atherosclerosis; 2. Low Density Lipo-protein (LDL) which promotes atherosclerosis.

COMPLEX CARBOHYDRATES Carbohydrates occurring in an unprocessed form, and complexed with fibre, minerals and other nutrients. They are more slowly absorbed and utilized than processed or refined carbohydrates.

CORTISONE A steroid hormone made by the adrenal glands and also synthetically in laboratories. It improves well-being and has a powerful anti-inflammatory effect.

DIURETIC A substance, whether synthetic or natural, which stimulates the kidneys to excrete salt (sodium chloride) and water, thereby relieving fluid retention.

ENDOCRINE GLANDS Glands that manufacture and secrete hormones.

ENDOCRINOLOGY The study and treatment of disorders of the glands and the hormones they secrete.

ENDOMETRIOSIS The presence of endometrium (which is normally confined inside the uterine cavity) outside of the uterus, scattered about inside the abdomen and pelvic cavities.

ENZYMES Proteins produced by living cells, which function as catalysts in specific biochemical reactions.

ESSENTIAL FATTY ACIDS Fatty acids necessary for cellular metabolism, which cannot be made by the body, but must be supplied in the diet. Suitable sources are oil of evening primrose, fish, fish oil, nuts, seeds and their oils.

ESTRADIOL A natural estrogen made by the ovaries. It is the most potent of all the natural estrogens.

ESTROGENS The female sex hormones secreted by the ovary being responsible for the female characteristics of breasts, feminine curves and menstruation.

EVENING PRIMROSE OIL The oil extracted from the beautiful evening primrose plant, which is renowned for its healing and tonifying properties. It is an excellent source of the omega 6 fatty acids, in particular the essential fatty acid known as gamma linolenic acid (GLA).

EXPECTORANT A substance that promotes the removal of mucus

from the respiratory tract.

FEMALE SEX HORMONES The two sex hormones produced by the female ovary—namely estrogen and progesterone.

FIBROIDS Non-cancerous growths of the uterus consisting of muscle and fibrous tissue.

'FRIENDLY PROGESTERONES' Those type of progesterones that exert a favorable effect upon our blood vessels and skin and do not increase cholesterol, promote weight gain or masculine changes in the skin. Examples are cyproterone acetate, gestodene or desogestrel.

GLANDS Organs or tissues, generally soft and fleshy in consistency, that manufacture and secrete or excrete hormones that exert their effect elsewhere in the body.

GYNECOLOGY Study of diseases of reproductive organs in women.

GYNECOLOGICAL ENDOCRINOLOGY Study of the hormones produced by women. It is a relatively new medical specialty which is expanding rapidly and brings the promise of exciting new developments and hope for many women.

HIRSUTISM A condition of excessive facial and body hair, excluding the scalp.

HORMONES Chemicals produced by various glands, which are then transported around the body.

HORMONE REPLACEMENT THERAPY (HRT) The administration of hormonal preparations (natural or synthetic) to replace the loss of natural hormones produced by various glands.

HYPOTHALAMUS A major centre situated at the base of the brain, regulating body temperature, thirst, appetite and other hormonal glands. It releases hormones that travel directly to the pituitary gland via a stalk.

IMMUNE SYSTEM The defence and surveillance system of the body, which protects against infection by micro-organisms and invasion by foreign proteins.

INFLAMMATION A condition characterised by swelling, redness, heat and pain in any tissue as a result of trauma, irritation, infection or imbalances in immune function.

INFUSION The process of steeping or soaking in a liquid to extract medicinal properties without boiling.

ISOTONIC Having equal tension or tone.

LYMPHATIC SYSTEM Drains fluid from the tissue spaces, transports fats and assists with immunity and our ability to overcome disease.

MALE HORMONE A hormone which promotes characteristics in the body such as facial and body hair, balding, acne, deepening of the voice and increased libido.

MENOPAUSE The final cessation of menstruation. The last period.

MENSTRUAL CYCLE The period of time from the first day of menstruation to the first day of the next menstruation.

METABOLIC RATE The rate at which the body converts food energy into kinetic energy.

METABOLISM Chemical processes utilising the raw materials of nutrients, oxygen and vitamins along with enzymes to produce energy for bodily functions.

NATUROPATHIC MEDICINE The treatment of illness with naturally occurring substances such as organic foods, juices, nutritional supplements and herbs.

NON-ANDROGENIC Not causing masculine effects in the body.

NUTRIENT A nutritious substance or component of food.

OFFAL Parts of a butchered animal usually regarded as worthless, i.e. organ meats.

ORAL Denoting a drug to be taken by mouth.

OSTEOPOROSIS Loss of bone mass due to loss of bone minerals. Skeletal atrophy. Porous condition of bones.

OVARIES The female sex glands (gonads) located on each side of the uterus, which produce eggs and the female sex hormones (estrogen and progesterone).

PITUITARY GLAND A mushroom-shaped gland connected by a vascular stalk to the base of the brain. The pituitary gland manufactures hormones, which in turn control other hormonal glands, such as the thyroid, adrenals, ovaries, testicles and breasts.

POLYCYSTIC OVARIAN SYNDROME A condition of hormonal imbalance characterised by excessive male hormones and irregular menstruation. It is strongly inherited and may be triggered by stress or weight gain.

POLYCYSTIC OVARIES The type of ovaries present in women with the Polycystic Ovarian Syndrome. They have more than ten small follicles per ovary aligned around the edge of the ovary, whereas in a 'normal' ovary they are distributed more evenly throughout the ovary.

They can be seen by an ultrasound scan of the pelvis.

PRE-MENOPAUSAL The years, generally four to five, leading up to the menopause, characterized by a time of hormonal imbalance.

PROGESTOGENS Synthetic forms of the natural female hormone progesterone. They are commonly used in the OCP and HRT and regulate menstrual bleeding. Examples are norethisterone, norgestrel and medroxy-progesterone acetate.

PROSTAGLANDINS Chemicals manufactured throughout the body which exert a hormone-like effect and influence muscular contraction, circulation and inflammation.

PSYCHOTHERAPY The treatment of mental and emotional imbalance through analysis of the thought processes, defence mechanisms and subconscious mind.

SEX HORMONES The male and female hormones produced by the testicles, ovaries, adrenal glands and fat, e.g. estrogen, testosterone and progesterone.

STEROID DRUGS AND HORMONES This group of hormones have a ring-like chemical structure. Examples of steroid hormones are cortisone and the male and female sex hormones.

SUBCUTANEOUS LAYER The fatty layer of tissue lying immediately underneath the skin.

SYNERGISTIC NUTRIENT A nutrient which helps or increases the effect of other body nutrients.

TANNIN Tannic Acid—an astringent compound.

TESTOSTERONE The major male sex hormone.

THYROID GLAND The endocrine gland situated in front of the neck which produces the hormone thyroxine.

TOFU Bean curd.

TONIC Producing and restoring normal tone and having the power to invigorate.

UTERUS The womb.

ULTRASOUND SCAN A method of visualising the internal organs, foetus and blood vessels. Ultrasound does not incur any radiation exposure and utilises very high frequency sound waves (more than 20 000 hertz) that are above the audible limit.

CHAPTER TEN

METABOLISM AND CELLULITE

How can I Boost My Metabolism and Banish Cellulite?

Cellulite is a stubborn problem for many people and is far more common in women. Even women who are not overweight may suffer with cellulite. If you have cellulite do not become depressed as it can gradually be eliminated by easy and proven techniques to improve your metabolism. Cellulite is the term used to describe the build up of irregular, lumpy fat deposits typically around the buttocks, hips and thighs. Cellulite has an "orange peel" appearance because the overlying skin is dimpled. The key to eradicating cellulite and keeping it off is found in restoring a healthy metabolism!

What is metabolism?

Metabolism is the term used to describe the inner chemical processes of the cells during which food energy is turned into cellular energy.

The rate at which this happens is called the metabolic rate. If you have a high metabolic rate your cells will convert food energy into cellular energy quickly, which means that you will not gain weight easily. Conversely if you have a low metabolic rate, you will not convert food energy into cellular energy efficiently and food energy will be stored in the form of body fat. It is well recognized that metabolism has a lot to do with excessive weight gain and those with a slow or sluggish metabolism will gain weight very easily and tend to develop cellulite. Fat cells in areas of cellulite have a very low metabolic rate and this is why it is so hard to burn fat off from these affected areas.

What Controls the Metabolic Rate?

A. The Liver

A healthy liver is the major fat burning organ in the body and regulates fat metabolism in several very sophisticated ways. In simple terms we can describe the liver as an organ which can burn unwanted body fat, or pump excessive fat out of the body through the bile into the intestines.

Many people who develop cellulite have an underlying problem with their liver function. In such cases the liver has turned from a fat burner into a fat storer, and we see fatty deposits building up in the liver itself. It is as if the liver has become a warehouse for fat.

Improving the liver function is essential to eradicate cellulite.

B. The Thyroid Gland

The thyroid gland produces the hormone called thyroxine, also known as T4. Thyroxine is not an active hormone and must be converted inside the body cells to its active form called Triiodothyronine or T3.

T3 acts directly upon the energy factories inside the cells (mitochondria), to speed up the rate at which they convert food energy into physical energy. In other words T3 speeds up the metabolic rate.

The thyroid gland can be considered to be the throttle or accelerator of body metabolism.

The conversion of T4 into T3 can slow down with advancing years, poor diet, or exposure to various toxins such as excessive alcohol or insecticides. This is called "thyroid resistance" and results in abnormally low levels of T3. People with low levels of T3 will have a very slow metabolic rate and will age more rapidly. They will experience fluid retention, dryness of the skin and hair, easy weight gain and a tendency to puffy cellulite. It is easy to check the levels of the T4 and T3 hormones with a simple blood test that your local doctor can arrange.

Factors that increase Cellulite

- Sluggish metabolic rate caused by imbalances in the function of the thyroid gland and liver.
- Build up of toxins in the fat cells. These toxins overload the energy factories inside the fat cells, which reduces their ability to burn fat. Most of these toxins are fat-soluble and only the liver can turn fat soluble toxins into water-soluble toxins. If this does not occur the toxins cannot be eliminated from the body and will stay inside the fat cells. This will lead to persistence of cellulite.
- Hormonal changes which occur during pregnancy and the premenstrual phase of the cycle. Many women complain of weight gain and increased cellulite before menstrual bleeding, and during and after pregnancy. This can be prevented by correct diet and keeping your metabolism at efficient levels.
- Lack of exercise, which will reduce blood supply to the fatty areas and increase fluid retention in cellulite areas. We recommend swimming, cycling and brisk walking.
- Eating the wrong types of fats, which increases the workload of the

liver. These "heavy fats" tend to accumulate inside the fat cells causing the cells to become hard and swollen. It is as if these fat cells become choked with fat, which slows down the metabolic processes inside the fat cells. These hard swollen fat cells then become trapped by connective tissues, which makes them irregular and lumpy in appearance. This gives the appearance of cellulite. It is vital to avoid these "heavy fats" if you want to eradicate cellulite.

The fats to avoid are found in:
Deep Fried foods
Processed foods and snack foods containing hydrogenated vegetable oils
Fatty parts of animal meats
Chicken skin and pork crackling
Preserved meats such as ham, bacon, sausage, pizza meats, etc
Smoked meats and delicatessen meats
Margarine and oils that are not cold pressed
Dairy products (milk, butter, cheese, cream, chocolate, icecream and yoghurt)
Foods containing dairy products as additives

To avoid these types of fats may necessitate quite a few changes in your diet, however you will find that this is easy to stick to. The good news is that you will not be hungry while avoiding these fatty foods because you will be able to eat and enjoy the good fats which are the "light fats". The good fats will give you a feeling of fullness and satisfaction while boosting energy and enhancing metabolism. The good fats are known as essential fatty acids and have not been processed in any way. They must be fresh to be beneficial for health.

Examples of foods containing the good fats are:
Cold pressed seed and vegetable oils
Raw nuts and seeds
Legumes (beans, peas, lentils)
Seafood (fresh or canned)
Spirulina, evening primrose oil, borage oil, lecithin
Many fruits and vegetables, especially egg plant, bananas and green-leafy vegetables.
Nut and seed spreads (eg. tahini, almond paste, and hummus)
Eggs in moderation (say around 8 per week) are safe. These are allowed because although they contain some cholesterol, it is combined with lecithin and sulfur bearing amino acids,which help the liver to burn fat. If you want to eradicate cellulite obtain your fats from our list of good

fats, and avoid the "hard fats" in the first list. You will be surprised just how easy and effective this is. The essential fatty acids found in the "good fat foods" will keep your fat cells soft and flexible and give them healthy cell membranes. This will enhance energy flow inside and across the cell membranes, which will keep the metabolic rate inside the fat cells at a high level. This will prevent the fat cells from becoming swollen and hard with excessive fats. Your fat cells will remain soft, flexible and of normal size, and therefore cellulite cannot develop.

Your Body Type and Cellulite
There are 4 different body types:
Android, Gynaeoid, Thyroid and Lymphatic *(see below)*

These 4 body types have unique hormonal and metabolic characteristics. Some body types gain weight easily and are also more susceptible to cellulite. In all body types the above guidelines concerning the good (light) fats and the bad (heavy) fats can be followed to eradicate cellulite. The supplements discussed to enhance fat burning and metabolism will be effective for cellulite in all the body types because they work on the cellular level.

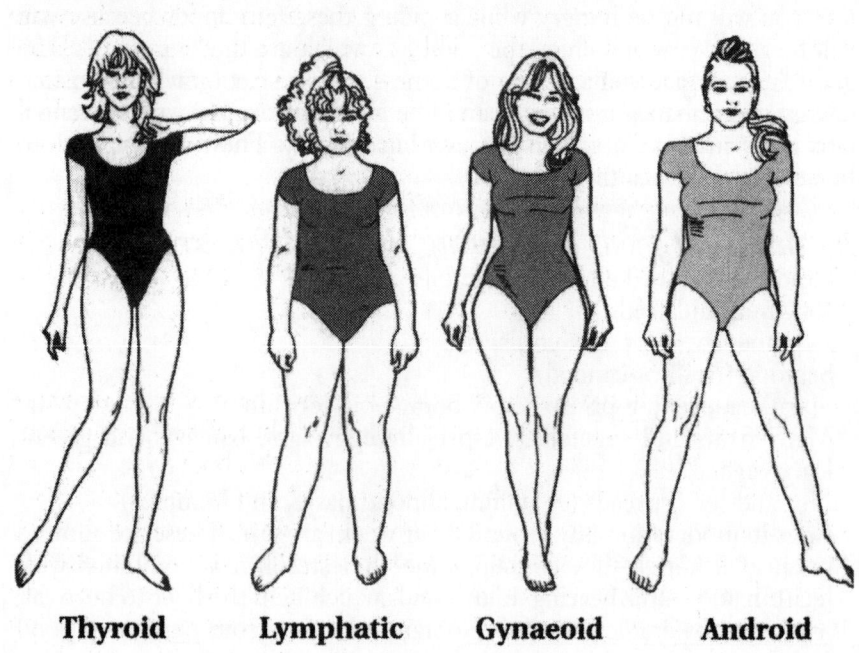

| **Thyroid** | **Lymphatic** | **Gynaeoid** | **Android** |

Android Type

The Android body type has broad shoulders and strong muscular limbs. The trunk is somewhat straight up and down and there is not much of a waist. The pelvis is narrow and the hips do not flare. Android types have an anabolic metabolism, which means that they tend to be "body-building" and will gain weight in the upper part of their body so that they may become apple-shaped. Most of their weight gain occurs on the front of the abdomen. They build muscle mass easily and make good athletes. They tend to produce more male hormones than do the other body types. Android types tend to crave foods that are high in cholesterol and salt. The body turns cholesterol into steroid hormones, which will have a body building effect. This may lead to some cellulite in the abdominal area, trunk and upper buttocks, but not below the hips.

Gynaeoid Type

The Gynaeoid body type is the curvy shape with small to medium shoulders tapering to a small waist and then flaring below to wide curvaceous hips. Weight gain occurs only on the thighs and lower buttocks and gives a very feminine and curvy shape. Many gynaeoid types will have a big problem with cellulite accumulating around the upper thighs and buttocks. If they try to lose weight with just any old low-fat low-calorie diet, it can be quite frustrating because weight will tend to come off easily from areas where there is not a problem, while the thighs and buttocks retain their fatty deposits and cellulite. They often have a hormonal imbalance called "estrogen dominance" which means that there is too much estrogen compared to progesterone. They often crave foods combining high amounts of fat and sugar, which will increase their sensitivity to estrogen, leading to more cellulite in the buttocks and thighs.

They do well with plant hormones (phytoestrogens), which have a balancing effect and help them to reduce their estrogen dependent weight gain. A suitable product for women wanting phytoestrogens is FemmePhase.

Thyroid Type

The Thyroid body type is characterised by a fine narrow bone structure and long limbs. This body type often has a "race-horse" or "grey hound" appearance. Many dancers and models belong to this body type. Thyroid types often crave stimulants such as caffeine, nicotine and artificial sweeteners, and may miss meals. They often have problems with unstable blood sugar levels, which can cause fatigue and cravings for sugar and stimulants. Generally speaking, thyroid types do not gain weight easily and have a very high metabolic rate. Of all the body types they are least likely to develop cellulite and if it does occur, it is on the buttocks and back of the thighs.

Lymphatic Types

Lymphatic body types gain weight all over the body, and have a "cuddly baby doll" appearance. Weight gain occurs very easily because lymphatic types have a very low metabolic rate. They also have a dysfunctional lymphatic system resulting in generalised fluid retention, which makes them look fatter than they are. They are prone to deposits of fat swollen with lymphatic fluid, which can cause severe cellulite. This type of cellulite gives them thick puffy limbs so that it is hard to see their bone structure. They often avoid exercise and crave dairy products, both of which will exacerbate their cellulite.

In The Past

Years ago it was recognised that there were different body types and they were categorised according to their shape only. This was before we understood the hormonal and metabolic differences between the body types. For your interest, just in case you find them in some old textbook I will describe them for you.

Android	was called the mesomorph
Thyroid	was called the ectomorph
Lymphatic	was called the endomorph
Gynaeoid	this body type was not described, probably being considered a combination of several types.

Natural Supplements to Help Metabolism

These will stimulate fat burning and reduce cellulite.

A. Improve Liver Function

This will increase the ability of the liver to burn fat and pump fat out of the body through the bile. It will also help to breakdown fat-soluble toxins that would otherwise become trapped in the fatty tissues and lead to cellulite. Liver tonics are the most effective strategy, however you will need a powerful tonic that can really improve liver function. I recommend a liver tonic called Livatone Plus that contains B vitamins , anti-oxidants, green tea, zinc, lecithin, cruciferous vegetable powder, and the amino acids taurine, cysteine, glutamine, and glycine, plus the powerful liver herb called Milk Thistle. Dosage is half a teaspoon mixed in juice twice daily or two capsules twice daily. Eat raw fruits and vegetables with every meal and drink at least 8 glasses (2litres/4 pints) of filtered water everyday.

B. Improve Thyroid Function

The thyroid gland has a high requirement for trace minerals because the enzymes that produce thyroid hormone (T4) and convert it to the active form (T3) are dependent upon trace minerals. The most important minerals for this process are selenium, zinc, manganese and iodine. Many people with cellulite have a deficiency of trace minerals, which leads to sluggish thyroid function and a low metabolic rate. To boost trace minerals I recommend that you include in the diet unprocessed grains, nuts, seeds and legumes.

I have found that an excellent way to boost trace minerals needed by the thyroid gland, is to take Selenomune powder enhanced with these minerals. It is a food supplement that contains an easily absorbed form of organic minerals. Selenomune contains selenium, chromium, molybdenum, zinc, manganese, magnesium, calcium, vegetable powders (also high in trace minerals), and the herb kelp (very high in trace minerals). Selenomune also contains the natural ingredient (usually extracted from apples) called Malic acid, which helps the cells to turn food energy into physical energy. Generally speaking you will require two teaspoons of this powder daily to obtain these benefits. Stir the powder into juice and take with meals.

C. Stimulate your Fat Cells to Burn Fat

These natural substances will help you to burn fat safely without drug induced side effects. They are all combined together in a tablet called METABOCEL. Each tablet of Metabocel contains:

- Tyrosine.
- Brindleberry - (Garcinia quaesita) (extra strength) which is the richest source of Hydroxy Citric Acid (HCA).
- Kelp .
- Vitamin B6.
- Zinc amino acid chelate, chromium picolinate and capsicum extract are able to enhance the effect of tyrosine and brindleberry.

Actions: Natural substances, which eliminate cellulite and reduce weight scientifically, must be able to do the following:

Stimulate thyroid function
Stimulate brown fat metabolism
Reduce sugar cravings
Stabilize blood sugar levels
Boost energy

Tyrosine is a precursor of the energy hormones thyroxine and adrenalin. Tyrosine stimulates thyroid gland function and therefore metabolism. Tyrosine is needed by the thyroid gland to manufacture thyroid hormones. It reduces brain fatigue and improves mood.

Kelp is a sea herb and is an excellent source of trace minerals, especially iodine, which is required to make thyroid hormone. Kelp contains many trace minerals needed by the body and is an excellent aid to general health. Kelp contains organic iodine and is not a problem for those allergic to inorganic iodine. It is beneficial for the glandular system, especially the thyroid, pituitary and adrenal glands.

Brindleberry is a fruit used for centuries by the people of Asia because it enhances the flavor and satisfaction of meals. The rind of this fruit is rich in Hydroxy Citric Acid (HCA). Brindleberry is more effective if it is combined with tyrosine, kelp, vitamin B6, zinc, chromium and capsicum as found in METABOCEL.

HCA is proven to naturally suppress the appetite and stop the production of new fat. HCA from Brindleberry is clinically proven to help inhibit the production of fat by blocking the enzyme that causes fat to be stored by the body. So while your losing weight you are also halting the formation of new fat..

All these natural ingredients are available combined together in METABOCEL. For more information on natural fat burning nutrients phone Dr Cabot's Health Line on 1888 75 LIVER or visit www.weightcontroldoctor.com

Avoid artificial stimulants, artificial sweeteners, amphetamine type drugs and the herb Ephedra, because these things will temporarily hype up your metabolic rate and reduce your appetite. However once you stop them your system has become dependent upon them and you will probably feel tired, depressed and very hungry. The worst thing of all is that when you come off these stimulants your metabolic rate will be temporarily lower than ever and you will gain weight rapidly.

The natural fat burners that I have discussed have a balancing effect upon the overall metabolism. They will not cause any dramatic changes in your metabolic rate, which is good, otherwise you will become a yoyo dieter and will get bigger over the long term.

If you have queries concerning your weight, body type, metabolism or cellulite, why not phone us at Dr Cabot's Health Line on 1888 75 LIVER.

We have a nutritionist called Susie Clift who works closely with Dr Sandra Cabot and is committed to your weight control program. Susie is excellent for people of all ages, including children battling with a weight problem. You can email Susie Clift with your weight control questions. VISIT OUR WEB SITE – www.weightcontroldoctor.com which has an interactive questionnaire to work out your body type – you will enjoy this exercise!

INDEX

Numbers in *italic* denote illustrations